Medieval Medicine

James J. Walsh

Table of Contents

CHAPTER I 5
CHAPTER II 14
CHAPTER III 22
CHAPTER IV 34
CHAPTER V 41
CHAPTER VI 48
CHAPTER VII 58
CHAPTER VIII 73
CHAPTER IX 82
CHAPTER X 90
HAPTER XI 99
APPENDIX I 110
APPENDIX II 113

CHAPTER I

INTRODUCTORY

To understand the story of Medieval Medicine, the reader must recall briefly the course of Roman history. Rome, founded some eight centuries before Christ, was at first the home of a group of adventurers who, in the absence of women enough to supply wives for their warriors, went out and captured the maidens of a neighbouring Sabine town. The feud which broke out as a result was brought to an end by the women now become the wives of the Romans, and an alliance was made. Gradually Rome conquered the neighbouring cities, but was ever so much more interested in war and conquest than in the higher life. The Etruscan cities, which came under her domination, now reveal in their ruins art objects of exquisite beauty and the remains of a people of high artistic culture. When Rome conquered Carthage, Carthage was probably the most magnificent city in the world, and Rome was a very commonplace collection of houses. Culture did not come to Rome until after her conquest of Greece, when "captive Greece led her captor captive."

Sir Henry Maine's expression that whatever lives and moves in the intellectual life is Greek in origin may not be unexceptionably true, but it represents a generalization of very wide application.

Rome was stimulated in art and architecture and literature by touch with the Greeks, and her own achievements, important though they were, were little better than copies of Greek originals. The Romans themselves acknowledged this very frankly. When in the course of time the barbarian nations from the North and West of Europe came down in large numbers into Italy, and finally gained control of the Roman Empire, they had but very little interest in the Greek sources, and decadence of the intellectual life was inevitable. This was particularly true as regards scientific subjects, and above all for medicine; for the Romans had always depended on Greek physicians, and Galen in the second century, like Alexander of Tralles in the seventh, represent terms in the series of physicians who reached distinction at Rome.

The key to the history of medicine in the Middle Ages, then, is always the presence of Greek influence. This persisted in the Near East, and consequently serious scientific medicine continued to flourish there, at first among the Christians and later among the Arabs. It was not for any special incentive of their own that the Arabs became the intellectual leaders of Europe during the tenth and eleventh centuries, but the fact that their geographical position in Asia Minor close to Greek sources provided them with the opportunity to know the old

Greek authors, especially in philosophy and medicine, and therefore to be almost forced to become the channels through which Greek influences were carried into the West once more.

Before the coming of the Arabs, however—that is, before the rise of Mohammedanism—there was an important chapter of medieval medicine which is often not appreciated at its true worth. The contributors to it deserve to be well known, and fortunately for us in the modern time were properly appreciated during the early days of the art of printing, in the Renaissance time, and accordingly their books were printed, and came to be distributed in many copies, which have rendered them readily available in the modern time.

In Asia Minor, where Greek influence persisted as it did not in Italy, we have a series of distinguished contributors to medicine, or rather, medical literature—that is, men whose books represent a valuable compilation and digestion of the important medical writings from before their time, often enriched by their own experience. The first of these was Aëtios Amidenus—that is, Aëtios of Amida—born in the town of that name in Mesopotamia on the Upper Tigris (now Diarbekir), who flourished in the sixth century. Aëtios, or in the Latin form Aëtius, wrote a textbook that has often been republished in the modern time, and that shows very clearly how well the physicians of this period faced their medical and surgical problems, how thoroughly equipped they were by faithful study of the old Greek writers, and how successfully they coped with the difficulties of the cases presented to them. He is eminently conservative, a careful observer, who uses all the means at his command and who well deserves the interest that has been manifested in him at many periods during the almost millennium and a half elapsed since his death.

After Aëtius came Alexander of Tralles, from another of these towns of Asia Minor that we would consider insignificant, sometimes termed Trallianus for this reason. He must be reputed one of the great independent thinkers in medicine whose writings have deservedly attracted attention not only in his own time, but long afterwards in the Renaissance period, and with whose works everyone who cares to know anything about the development of medical history must be familiar. One detail of his life has always seemed to me to correct a whole series of misapprehensions with regard to the earlier Middle Ages. Alexander was one of five brothers, all of whose names have come down to us through nearly 1,500 years because of what they accomplished at the great Capital of the East. The eldest of them was Anthemios, the architect of the great Church of Santa Sophia. A second brother was Methrodoros, a distinguished grammarian and teacher at Constantinople. A third brother was a prominent jurist in the Imperial Courts of the capital; while a fourth brother, Dioscoros, was, like Alexander, a physician of repute, but remained in his birthplace Tralles, and acquired a substantial practice there.

There is sometimes the feeling that at this time in the world's history, the end of the sixth and the beginning of the seventh century, men had but little initiative, and above all very little power of achievement in the intellectual order. Anyone who knows Santa Sophia in Constantinople, however, will recognize at once that the architect who conceived and superintended the construction of that great edifice was a genius of a high order, not lacking in initiative, but on the contrary possessed of a wonderful power of original accomplishment. No greater constructive work, considering all the circumstances, has perhaps ever been successfully planned and executed. It would scarcely be expected that the brother of the man who conceived and finished Santa Sophia would, if he set out to write a textbook of medicine, make an egregious failure of it. Surely his work would not be all unworthy of his brother's reputation, and the family genius should lift him up to important accomplishment. This is literally what we find true with regard to Alexander. After years of travel which led him into Italy, Gaul, Spain, and Africa, he settled down at Rome, and practised medicine successfully until a very old age, and probably lectured there, for some of his books are in the form of lectures.

Fortunately for us, he committed his knowledge and his experience to writing, which has come down to us.

A third of these greater writers on medicine in the early Middle Ages was Paul of Ægina—Æginetus as he is sometimes known. There has been some question as to his date in history, but as he quotes Alexander of Tralles there seems to be no doubt now that his career must be placed in the first half of the seventh century. We shall see more of him, as also of his great contemporaries and predecessors of the early Middle Ages, Aëtios and Alexander of Tralles, in a subsequent chapter. Besides these men who were known for their writings, a series of less known Christian physicians were praised by their contemporaries for their knowledge of medicine. Among them are particularly to be noted certain members of an Arabian family with the title Bachtischua, a name which is derived from the Arabic words *Bocht Jesu*—that is, servant of Jesus—who, having studied among the Greek Christians in the cities of Asia Minor, were called to the Court of Haroun al-Raschid and introduced Greek medicine to the Mohammedans. I have pointed out in my volume "Old-Time Makers of Medicine"[1] that "it was their teaching which aroused Moslem scholars from the apathy that characterized the attitude of the Arabian people towards science at the beginning of Mohammedanism."

After this preliminary period of early medieval medical development, the next important phase of medicine and surgery in the Middle Ages developed in the southern part of Italy at Salerno. Here came the real awakening from that inattention to intellectual interests which characterized Italy after the invasion of the northern barbarians. The reason for the early Renaissance in this neighbourhood is not far to seek. In the older times Sicily had been a Greek colony, and the southern portion of Italy had been settled by Greeks and came to be known as Magna Græcia. The Greek language continued to be spoken in many parts even during the earlier medieval centuries, and Greek never became the utterly unknown tongue it was in Northern Italy. With the turning of attention to education in the later Middle Ages, the Southern Italians were brought almost at once in contact with Greek sources, and the earlier Renaissance began. With this in mind, it is comparatively easy to understand the efflorescence of culture in Southern Italy, and the development of the important University of Salerno and its great accomplishment, particularly in scientific matters, though all this came almost entirely as a consequence of the opportunity for Greek influence to have its effect there.

It is sometimes said that Arabian influence meant much for the development of Salerno, and that it was because the southern part of the Italian peninsula was necessarily rather closely in touch with Arabian culture that an early awakening took place down there. The Mohammedans occupied so many of the islands of the Mediterranean, as well as Spain, that their influence was felt deeply all along its shore, and hence the first university of Europe in modern times came into existence in this part of the world. Montpellier is sometimes, though not so often, said to have had the same factor in its early development. Undoubtedly there was some Arabian influence in the foundation of Salerno. The oldest traditions of the University show this rather clearly. This Arabian influence, however, has been greatly exaggerated by some modern historical writers. Led by the thought that Christianity was opposed to culture, and above all to science, they were quite willing to suggest any other influences than Christian as the source of so important a movement in the history of human progress as Salerno proved to be. The main influence at Salerno, however, was Greek, and the proof of this is, as insisted by Gurlt in his "History of Surgery," that the great surgeons of Salerno do not refer to Arabian sources, but to Greek authors, and their books do not show traces of Arabian influences, but on the contrary have many Græcisms in them.

Salerno represents an especially important chapter in the history of Medieval Medicine. As we shall see, the teachers at the great medical school there set themselves in strenuous opposition to the Arabian tendency to polypharmacy, by which the Oriental mind had seriously hurt medicine, and what is still more to the credit of these Salernitan teachers, they developed surgery far beyond anything that the Arabs had attempted. Indeed, surgery in the later centuries of Arabian influence had been distinctly neglected, but enjoyed a great revival at Salerno. Besides, the Salernitan physicians used all the natural methods of cure, air, water, exercise, and diet, very successfully. If any other proof were needed that Arabian influence was not prominent at Salerno, surely it would be found in the fact that women physicians enjoyed so many privileges there. This is so entirely opposed to Mohammedan ways as to be quite convincing as a demonstration of the absence of Arabian influence.

From Salerno, the tradition of medicine and surgery spread to Bologna early in the thirteenth century, and thence to the other universities of Italy and to France. Montpellier represented an independent focus of modern progress in medicine, partly due to close relationship with the Moors in Spain and the Greek influences they carried with them from Asia Minor, but not a little of it consequent upon the remnants of the older Greek culture, still not entirely dead even in the thirteenth century, because Marseilles, not far away, had been a Greek colony originally, and still retained living Greek influence, and wherever Greek got a chance to exercise its stimulant incentive modern scientific medicine began to develop.

France owed most of her development in medicine and surgery at the end of the Middle Ages to the stream of influence that flowed out of Italian universities. Such men as Lanfranc, who was an Italian born but exiled; Mondeville, who studied in Italy; and Guy de Chauliac, who has so freely acknowledged his obligation to Italian teachers, were the capital sources of medical and surgical teaching in France in the later Middle Ages.

It is thus easy to see how the two periods of historical import in medicine at the beginning and end of the Middle Ages may be placed in their intimate relation to Greek influences. At the beginning, Greek medicine was not yet dead in Asia Minor, and it influenced the Arabs. When the revival came, it made itself first felt in the portions of Southern Italy and Southern France where Greek influence had been strongest and still persisted. Fortunately for us, the great Renaissance printers and scholars, themselves touched by the Greek spirit of their time, put the books of the writers of these two periods into enduring printed form, and in more recent years many reprints of them have been issued. These volumes make it possible for us to understand just how thoroughly these colleagues of the Middle Ages faced their problems, and solved them with a practical genius that deserves the immortality that their works have been given.

The history of medicine and surgery during the Middle Ages has been greatly obscured by the assumption that at this time scientific medicine and surgery could scarcely have developed because men were lacking in the true spirit of science. The distinction between modern and medieval education is often said to be that the old-time universities sought to increase knowledge by deduction, while the modern universities depend on induction. Inductive science is often said to be the invention of the Renaissance period, and to have had practically no existence during the Middle Ages. The medieval scholars are commonly declared to have preferred to appeal to authority, while modern investigators turn to experience. Respect for authority is often said to have gone so far in the Middle Ages that no one ventured practically to assert anything unless he could find some authority for it. On the other hand, if there was any acknowledged authority, say Aristotle or Galen, men so hesitated to contradict him that they usually followed one another like sheep, quoting their favourite author and swearing by the authority of their chosen master. Indeed, many modern writers have not hesitated to express the greatest possible wonder that the men of the Middle Ages did not think more for themselves, and above all did not trust to their own observation, rather than constantly rest under the shadow of authority.

Above all, it is often asked why there was no nature study in the Middle Ages—that is, why men did not look around them and see the beauties and the wonders of the world and of nature, and becoming interested in them, endeavour to learn as much as possible about them. Anyone who thinks that there was no nature study in the Middle Ages, however, is quite ignorant of the books of the Middle Ages. Dante, for instance, is full of the knowledge of nature. What he knows about the ants, and the bees, and many other insects; about the flowers, and the birds, and the habits of animals; about the phosphorescence at sea and the cloud effects, and nearly everything else in the world of nature around him, adds greatly to the interest of his poems. He uses all these details of information as figures in his "Divine Comedy," not in order to display his erudition, but to bring home his meaning with striking concreteness by the metaphors which he employs. There is probably no poet in the modern time who knows more about the science of his time than Dante, or uses it to better advantage.

It is sometimes thought that the medieval scholars did not consider that experience and observation were of any value in the search for truth, and that therefore there could have been no development of science. In an article on "Science at the Medieval Universities"[2] I made a series of quotations from the two great scientific scholars of the thirteenth century, Albertus Magnus and Roger Bacon, with regard to the question of the relative value of authority and observation in all that relates to physical science. Stronger expressions in commendation of observation and experiment as the only real sources of knowledge in such matters could scarcely be found in any modern scientist. In Albert's tenth book of his "Summa," in which he catalogues and describes all the trees, plants, and herbs known in his time, he declares: "All that is here set down is the result of our own experience, or has been borrowed from authors whom we know to have written what their personal experience has confirmed; for in these matters experience alone can be of certainty." In his impressive Latin phrase, *experimentum solum certificat in talibus*. With regard to the study of nature in general he was quite emphatic. He was a theologian as well as a scientist, yet in his treatise on "The Heavens and the Earth," he declared that: "In studying nature we have not to inquire how God the Creator may, as He freely wills, use His creatures to work miracles, and thereby show forth His power. We have rather to inquire what nature with its immanent causes can naturally bring to pass."

Roger Bacon, the recent celebration of whose seven hundredth anniversary has made him ever so much better known than before, furnishes a number of quotations on this subject. One of them is so strong that it will serve our purpose completely. In praising the work done by Petrus, one of his disciples whom we have come to know as Peregrinus, Bacon could scarcely say enough in praise of the thoroughly scientific temper, in our fullest sense of the term, of Peregrinus's mind. Peregrinus wrote a letter on magnetism, which is really a monograph on the subject, and it is mainly with regard to this that Roger Bacon has words of praise. He says: "I know of only one person who deserves praise for his work in experimental philosophy, for he does not care for the discourses of men and their wordy warfare, but quietly and diligently pursues the works of wisdom. Therefore, what others grope after blindly, as bats in the evening twilight, this man contemplates in their brilliancy, *because he is a master of experiment*. Hence, he knows all of natural science, whether pertaining to medicine and alchemy, or to matters celestial or terrestrial. He has worked diligently in the smelting of ores, as also in the working of minerals; he is thoroughly acquainted with all sorts of arms and implements used in military service and in hunting, besides which he is skilled in agriculture and in the measurement of lands. It is impossible to write a useful or correct treatise in experimental philosophy without mentioning this man's name. Moreover, he pursues knowledge for its own sake; for if he wished to obtain royal favour, he could easily find sovereigns who would honour and enrich him."

Roger Bacon actually wanted the Pope to forbid the study of Aristotle because his works were leading men astray from the true study of science—his authority being looked upon as so great that men did not think for themselves, but accepted his assertions. Smaller men are always prone to act thus at any period in the world's history, and we undoubtedly in our time have a very large number who do not think for themselves, but swear on the word of some master or other, and very seldom so adequate a master as Aristotle.

Bacon insisted that the four great grounds of human ignorance are: "First, trust in inadequate authority; second, that force of custom which leads men to accept without properly questioning what has been accepted before their time; third, the placing of confidence in the assertions of the inexperienced; and fourth, the hiding of one's own ignorance behind the parade of superficial knowledge, so that we are afraid to say, 'I do not know.'" Prof. Henry Morley suggested that: "No part of that ground has yet been cut away from beneath the feet of students, although six centuries have passed. We still make sheepwalks of second, third, and fourth, and fifth hand references to authority; still we are the slaves of habit, still we are found following too frequently the untaught crowd, still we flinch from the righteous and wholesome phrase, 'I do not know,' and acquiesce actively in the opinion of others that we know what we appear to know."

It used to be the custom to make little of the medieval scientists because of their reverence for Aristotle. Generations who knew little about Aristotle, especially those of the seventeenth and eighteenth centuries, were inclined to despise preceding generations who had thought so much of him. We have come to know more about Aristotle in our own time, however, and as a consequence have learned to appreciate better medieval respect for him. Very probably at the present moment there would be almost unanimous agreement of scholars in the opinion that Aristotle's was the greatest mind humanity has ever had. This is true not only because of his profound intellectual penetration, but above all because of the comprehensiveness of his intelligence. For depth and breadth of mental view on a multiplicity of subjects, Aristotle has never been excelled and has but very few rivals. The admiration of the Middle Ages for him, instead of being derogatory in any way to the judgment of the men of the time, or indicating any lack of critical appreciation, rather furnishes good reasons for high estimation of both these intellectual modes of the medieval mind. Proper appreciation of what is best is a much more difficult task than condemnation of what is less worthy of regard. It is the difference between constructive and destructive criticism. Medieval appreciation of Aristotle, then, constitutes rather a good reason for admiration of them than for depreciation of their critical faculty; and yet they never carried respect and reverence to unthinking worship, much less slavish adoration. Albertus Magnus, for instance, said: "Whoever believes that Aristotle was a God must also believe that he never erred; but if we believe that Aristotle was a man, then doubtless he was liable to err just as we are." We have a number of direct contradictions of Aristotle from Albert. A well-known one is that with regard to Aristotle's assertion that lunar rainbows appeared only twice in fifty years. Albert declared that he himself had seen two in a single year.

Galen, after Aristotle, was the author oftenest quoted in the Middle Ages, and most revered. Anyone who wants to understand this medieval reverence needs only to read Galen. There has probably never been a greater clinical observer in all the world than this Greek from Pergamos, whose works were destined to have so much influence for a millennium and a half after his time. How well he deserved this prestige only a careful study of his writings will reveal. It is simply marvellous what he had seen and writes about. Anatomy, physiology, pathological anatomy, diagnosis, therapeutics—all these were magnificently developed under his hands, and he has left a record of accurate and detailed observation. There are many absurdities easily to be seen in his writings now, but no one has yet written on medicine in any large way who has avoided absurdities, nor can anyone hope to, until we know much more of the medical sciences than at present. The therapeutics of any generation is always absurd to the second succeeding generation, it has been said. Those in the modern time who know their Galen best have almost as much admiration for him, in spite of all our advance in the knowledge of medicine, as the medieval people had. No wonder, seeing the depth and breadth of his knowledge, that he was thought so much of, and that men hesitated to contravene anything that he said.

Even in the authorities to which they turned with so much confidence, the medieval physicians are admirable. If man must depend on authority, then he could not have better than they had. As with regard to this, so in all other matters relating to the Middle Ages, the ordinarily accepted notions prove to have been founded on ignorance of actual details, and misconceptions as to the true significance of their point of view. To have contempt give way to admiration, we need only to know the realities even in such meagre details as can be given in a short manual of this kind. The thousand years of the Middle Ages are now seen to have been full of interesting and successful efforts in every mode of human activity, and medicine and surgery shared in this to the full.

CHAPTER II

EARLY MEDIEVAL MEDICINE

There are two distinct periods in the history of Medieval Medicine. The first concerns the early centuries, from the sixth to the ninth, and is occupied mainly with the contributions to medicine made by those who were still in touch with the old Greek writers; while the second represents the early Renaissance, when the knowledge of the Greek writers was gradually filtering back again, sometimes through the uncertain channel of the Arabic. Both periods contain contributions to medicine that are well worthy of consideration, and nearly always the writings that have been preserved for us demonstrate the fact that men were thinking for themselves as well as studying the Greek writers, and were making observations and garnering significant personal experience. The later Middle Ages particularly present material in this regard of far greater interest than was presumed to exist until comparatively recent historical studies were completed.

The real history of medicine in the Middle Ages—that is, of scientific medicine—is eclipsed by the story of popular medicine. So much has been said of the medical superstitions, many of which were rather striking, that comparatively little space has been left for the serious medical science and practice of the time, which contain many extremely interesting details. It is true that after the Crusades mummy was a favourite pharmacon, sometimes even in the hands of regular physicians; and *Usnea*, the moss from the skulls of the bodies of criminals that had been hanged and exposed in chains, was declared by many to be a sovereign remedy for many different ills; but it must not be forgotten that both of these substances continued to be used long after the medieval period, mummy even down to the middle of the eighteenth century, and Usnea almost as late. Indeed, it is probable that the seventeenth and eighteenth centuries present many more absurdities in therapeutics than do the later centuries of the Middle Ages. In this, as in so many other regards, the modern use of the adjective medieval has been symbolic of ignorance of the time rather than representative of realities in history. Popular medicine is always ridiculous, though its dicta are often accepted by supposedly educated people. This has always been true, however, and was never more true than in our own time, when the vagaries of medical faddism are so strikingly illustrated, and immense sums of money spent every year in the advertising of proprietary remedies, whose virtues are often sadly exaggerated, and whose tendency to work harm rather than good is thoroughly appreciated by all who know anything about medicine. The therapeutics of supposedly scientific medicine are often dubious enough. A distinguished French professor of physiology quoted, not long since, with approval, that characteristic French expression: "The therapeutics of any generation are always absurd to the second succeeding generation." When we look back on the abuse of calomel and venesection a century ago, and of the coal-tar derivatives a generation ago, and the overweening confidence in serums and vaccines almost in our own day, it is easy to understand that this law is still true. We can only hope that our generation will not be judged seven centuries from now by the remedies that were accepted for a time, and then proved to be either utterly ineffectual or even perhaps harmful to the patients to whom they were given.

When we turn our attention away from this popular pseudo-history of Medieval Medicine, which has unfortunately led so many even well-informed persons into entirely wrong notions with regard to medical progress during an important period, we find much that is of enduring interest. The first documents that we have in the genuine history of Medieval Medicine, after the references to the organizations of Christian hospitals at Rome and Asia Minor in the fourth and fifth centuries (see chapter Medieval Hospitals), are to be found in the directions provided in the rules of the religious orders for the care of the ailing. St. Benedict (480-543), the founder of the monks of the West, was particularly insistent on the thorough performance of this duty. The rule he wrote to guide his religious is famous in history as a great constitution of democracy, and none of its provisions are more significant than those which relate to the care of the health of members of the community.

One of the rules of St. Benedict required the Abbot to provide in the monastery an infirmary for the ailing, and to organize particular care of them as a special Christian duty. The wording of the rule in this regard is very emphatic. "The care of the sick is to be placed above and before every other duty, as if, indeed, Christ were being directly served in waiting on them. It must be the peculiar care of the Abbot that they suffer from no negligence. The Infirmarian must be thoroughly reliable, known for his piety and diligence and solicitude for his charge." The last words of the rule are characteristic of Benedict's appreciation of cleanliness as a religious duty, though doubtless also the curative effect of water was in mind. "Let baths be provided for the sick as often as they need them." As to what the religious infirmarians knew of medicine, at least as regards the sources of their knowledge and the authors they were supposed to have read, we have more definite information from the next historical document, that concerning medical matters in the religious foundation of Cassiodorus.

Cassiodorus (468-560), who had been the prime minister of the Ostrogoth Emperors, when he resigned his dignities and established his monastery at

Scillace in Calabria, was influenced deeply by St. Benedict, and was visited by the saint not long after the foundation.

His rule was founded on that of the Benedictines. Like that, it insisted especially on the care of the sick, and the necessity for the deep study of medicine on the part of those who cared for them. Cassiodorus laid down the law in this regard as follows: "I insist, brothers, that those who treat the health of the body of the brethren who have come into the sacred places from the world should fulfil their duties with exemplary piety. Let them be sad with others' suffering, sorrowful over others' dangers, sympathetic to the grief of those whom they have to care for, and always ready zealously to help others' misfortunes. Let them serve with sincere study to help those who are ailing as becomes their knowledge of medicine, and let them look for their reward from Him who can compensate temporal work by eternal wages. Learn, therefore, the nature of herbs, and study diligently the way to combine their various species for human health; but do not place your entire hope on herbs, nor seek to restore health only by human counsels. Since medicine has been created by God, and since it is He who gives back health and restores life, turn to Him. Remember, do all that you do in word or deed in the name of the Lord Jesus, giving thanks to God the Father through Him. And if you are not capable of reading Greek, read above all the translations of the Herbarium of Dioscorides, which describes with surprising exactness the herbs of the field. After this, read translations of Hippocrates and Galen, especially the Therapeutics, and Aurelius Celsus' 'De Medicina,' and Hippocrates' 'De Herbis et Curis,' and divers other books written on the art of medicine, which by God's help I have been able to provide for you in my library."

The monasteries are thus seen to have been in touch with Greek medicine from the earliest medieval time. The other important historical documents relating to Medieval Medicine which we possess concern the work of the men born and brought up in Asia Minor, for whom the Greeks were so close as to be living influences. Aëtius, Alexander of Tralles, and Paul of Ægina have each written a series of important chapters on medical subjects, full of interest because the writers knew their Greek classic medicine, and were themselves making important observations. Aëtius, for instance, had a good idea of diphtheria. He speaks of it in connection with other throat manifestations under the heading of "crusty and pestilent ulcers of the tonsils." He divides the anginas generally into four kinds. The first consists of inflammation of the fauces with the classic symptoms; the second presents no inflammation of the mouth nor of the fauces, but is complicated by a sense of suffocation—apparently our neurotic croup. The third consists of external and internal inflammation of the mouth and throat, extending towards the chin. The fourth is an affection rather of the neck, due to an inflammation of the vertebræ—retropharyngeal abscess—which may be followed by luxation, and is complicated by great difficulty of respiration. All of these have as a common symptom difficulty of swallowing. This is greater in one variety than in another at different times. In certain affections he remarks that even "drinks when taken are returned through the nose."

Aëtius declares quite positively that all the tumours of the neck region, with the exception of scirrhus, are easily cured, yielding either to surgery or to remedies. The exception is noteworthy. He evidently saw a good many of the functional disturbances and the enlargements of the thyroid gland, which are often so variable in character as apparently to be quite amenable to treatment, and which have actually been "cured" in the history of medicine by all sorts of things from the touch of the hangman's rope to the wrapping of the shed skin of the snake around the neck. A few cervical tumours were beyond resource. Aëtius suggests the connection between hypertrophy of the clitoris and certain exaggerated manifestations of the sexual instinct, as well as the development of vicious sexual habits.

It requires only a little study of this early medieval author to understand why Cornelius, at the time of the Renaissance, was ready to declare: "Believe me, that whoever is deeply desirous of studying things medical, if he would have the whole of Galen abbreviated and the whole of Orbiasius extended, and the whole of Paulus (of Ægina) amplified; if he would have all the special remedies of the old physicians, as well in pharmacy as in surgery, boiled down to a summa for all affections, he will find it in Aëtius."

Alexander of Tralles was, as we have said, the brother of the architect of Santa Sophia of Constantinople, and his writings on medical and surgical subjects are worthy of such a relationship. His principal work is a treatise on the "Pathology and Therapeutics of Internal Diseases" in twelve books, the first eleven books of which were evidently material gathered for lectures or teaching purposes. He treats of cough as a symptom due to hot or cold, dry or wet, dyscrasias. Opium preparations judiciously used he thought the best remedies, though he recommended also the breathing in of steam impregnated with various ethereal resins.

He outlines a very interesting because thoroughly modern treatment of consumption. He recommends an abundance of milk with a hearty nutritious diet, as digestible as possible. A good auxiliary to this treatment in his opinion was change of air, a sea voyage, and a stay at a watering-place. Ass's and mare's milk are much better for these patients than cow's and goat's milk. We realize now that there is not enough difference in the composition of these various milks to make their special prescription of physical importance, but it is probable that the suggestive influence of the taking of an unusual milk had a very favourable effect upon patients, and this effect was renewed with every drink taken, so that much good was ultimately accomplished. For hæmoptysis, especially when it was acute and due, as Alexander felt, to the rupture of a bloodvessel in the lungs, he recommended the opening of a vein at the elbow or the ankle—in order to divert the blood from the place of rupture to the healthy parts of the circulation. He insisted, however, that the patients must in addition rest, as well as take acid and astringent drinks, while cold compresses should be placed upon the chest [our ice-bags], and that they should take only a liquid diet, at most lukewarm, or, better, if agreeable to them, cold. When the bleeding stopped, he declared a milk cure [blood-maker] very useful for the restoration of these patients to their former strength.

He paid particular attention to diseases of the nervous system, and discussed headache at some length. Chronic or recurrent headache he attributed to diseases of the brain, plethora, biliousness, digestive disturbances, insomnia, and prolonged worry. Hemicrania he thought due to the presence of toxic materials, though it was also connected with abdominal disorders, especially in women. Alexander has much to say of the paralytic and epileptic conditions, and recommended massage, rubbings, baths, and warm applications for the former, and emphasized the need for careful directions as to the mode of life, and special attention to the gastro-intestinal tract, in the latter. A plain, simple diet, with regular bowels, he considers the most important basis for any successful treatment of epilepsy. Besides, he recommended baths, sexual abstinence, and regular exercise. He rejected treatment of the condition by surgery of the head, either by trephining or by incisions or by cauterization. His teaching is that of those who have had most experience with the disease in our own time. For sore throat he prescribes gargles or light astringents at the beginning, and stronger astringents, alum and soda dissolved in water, later in the case.

He particularly emphasized that trust should not be placed in any single method of treatment. Every available means of bringing relief to the patient should be tried. "The duty of the physician is to cool what is hot, to warm what is cold, to dry what is moist, and to moisten what is dry. He should look upon the patient as a besieged city, and try to rescue him with every means that art and science placed at his command. The physician should be an inventor, and think out new ways and means by which the cure of the patient's affection and the relief of his symptoms may be brought about." The most important factor in Alexander's therapeutics is his diet. Watering-places and various forms of mineral waters, as well as warm baths and sea baths, are constantly recommended by him. He took strong ground against the use of many drugs, and the rage for operating. The prophylaxis of disease is in Alexander's opinion the important part of the physician's duty. His treatment of fever shows the application of his principle: cold baths, cold compresses, and a cooling diet, were his favourite remedies. He encouraged diaphoresis nearly always, and gave wine and stimulating drugs when the patient was very weak.

Some of the general principles of medical practice which Alexander lays down are very significant even from our modern standpoint. He deprecated drastic remedies of all kinds. He did not believe in severe purgation nor in profuse or sudden blood-letting. His diagnosis was thorough and careful. He insisted particularly on inspection and palpation of the whole body; on careful examination of the urine, of the fæces, and the sputum; on study of the pulse and the breathing. He dwelt on the fact that much might be learned from the patient's history taken carefully. The general constitution was the most important element, in his estimation. His therapeutics is, above all, individual. Remedies must be administered with careful reference to the constitution, the age, the sex, and the condition of the patient's strength. Special attention must always be paid to seconding nature's efforts to cure. Alexander had no sympathy at all with the idea that nature was to be disturbed, much less that remedies must work in opposition to natural tendencies to recovery.

Paul of Ægina, educated at the University at Alexandria, probably flourished during the reign of the Emperor Heraclius, who died 641; his works contain more of surgical than of medical interest.

The Arab writer, Abul Farag, to whose references we owe the definite placing of the time when Paul lived, said that "he had special experience in women's diseases, and had devoted himself to them with great industry and success. The midwives of the time were accustomed to go to him and ask his counsel with regard to accidents that happen during and after parturition. He willingly imparted his information, and told them what they should do. For this reason he came to be known as the Obstetrician." Perhaps the term should be translated the man-midwife, for it was rather unusual for men to have much knowledge of this subject. His knowledge of the phenomena of menstruation was wide and definite. He knew a great deal of how to treat its disturbances. He seems to have been the first one to suggest that in metrorrhagia, with severe hæmorrhage from the uterus, the bleeding might be stopped by putting ligatures around the limbs. This same method has been suggested for severe hæmorrhage from the lungs as well as from the uterus in our own time. In hysteria he also suggested ligature of the limbs, and it is easy to understand that this might be a very strongly suggestive treatment for the severer forms of hysteria. It is possible, too, that the modification of the circulation to the nervous system induced by the shutting off of the circulation in large areas of the body might very well have a favourable physical effect in this affection. Paul's description of the use of the speculum is as complete as that in any modern textbook of gynæcology.

In the chapter on the medieval care of the insane, there are some clinical observations and suggestions as to treatment from Paul which make it very clear what a careful observer he was, and how rational in his application of such knowledge as he had to the treatment of patients. Probably his contributions to the difficult subject psychiatry, well above a thousand years ago, will serve to make his genius as a physician clearer than almost anything else that could be said of him.

Among the great Arabian physicians who represent the transition period, from the earlier Middle Ages directly under Greek influence, still surviving to the later Middle Ages, when the earlier Renaissance brought back the Greek masters once more, were Rhazes, Ali Abbas, Avicenna—whose name had been transformed from the Arabic Ibn Sina—Abulcasis, Avenzoar, and Averroes, the last named a philosophic theorist but not a physician. The first three named were born in the East, the last three in Spain. Besides these Maimonides, the great Jewish physician, who was born and educated at Cordova in Spain, deserves a place. In this earlier period Rhazes must be mentioned, while the others who merit special attention will be considered in the chapter on Later Medieval Medicine.

Rhazes (died 932) is one of the great epoch-makers in the history of medicine. He was the first to give us a clear description of smallpox. Some of his medical aphorisms are well worth noting, and make it very clear that he was a careful observer.

"When you can heal by diet, prescribe no other remedy; and where simple remedies suffice, do not take complicated ones."

Rhazes knew well the value of the influence of mind over body even in serious organic disease, and even though death seemed impending. One of his aphorisms is: "Physicians ought to console their patients even if the signs of impending death seem to be present." He considered the most valuable thing for the physician to do was to increase the patient's natural vitality. Hence his advice: "In treating a patient, let your first thought be to strengthen his natural vitality. If you strengthen that, you remove ever so many ills without more ado. If you weaken it, however, by the remedies that you use, you always work harm." The simpler the means by which the patient's cure can be brought about, the better in his opinion. He insists again and again on diet rather than artificial remedies. "It is good for the physician that he should be able to cure disease by means of diet, if possible, rather than by means of medicine." Another of his aphorisms seems worth while quoting: "The patient who consults a great many physicians is likely to have a very confused state of mind."

During the ninth and tenth centuries the Arabs continued to be the most important contributors to medicine, until the rise of the school at Salerno gave a new impetus to clinical observation, and furnished a new focus of medical attention in the West. Constantine brought whatever of Arab influence there was in Salerno, as we have pointed out in the chapter on the Beginnings of Medical Education; but after his time there is an originality about Salernitan medicine which makes it of great value as the foster-mother of the sciences related to medicine during the later Middle Ages.

CHAPTER III

SALERNO AND THE BEGINNINGS OF MODERN MEDICAL EDUCATION

The first medical school of modern history, and the institution which more than any other has helped us to understand the Middle Ages, is that of Salerno. Indeed, the accumulation of information with regard to this medical school, formally organized in the tenth century but founded a century earlier, and reaching a magnificent climax of development at the end of the twelfth century, has done more than anything else to revolutionize our ideas with regard to medieval education and the scientific interests of the Middle Ages. We owe this development of knowledge to De Renzi, whose researches with regard to matters Salernitan, and medical education generally in Italy in the Middle Ages, are well deserving of the prestige that has been at length accorded them.

In his "Storia della Medicina in Italia," published so modestly at Naples, the patient Italian student of medical history made an epoch-making contribution to the history of medicine. Unless one has actually read his book, it is difficult to understand how deep our obligations to him are. Anyone who might be tempted to think that medicine was not taken seriously, or that careful clinical observations and serious experiments for the cure of disease were not made at Salerno, will be amply undeceived by a reading of De Renzi. Above all, he makes it very clear that medical education was taken up with rigorous attention to details and high standards maintained. Three years of college work were demanded in preparation for medical studies, and then four years at medicine, followed by a year of practice with a physician, and even an additional year of special study in anatomy, had to be taken, if surgery were to be practised. All this before the licence to practise medicine was given; though the degree of doctor, granting the privilege of teaching as the word indicates, was conferred apparently after the completion of the four years at the medical school. We have had to climb back to these medieval standards of medical education in many countries in recent years, after a period of deterioration in which often the requirements for the physician's training for practice were ever so much lower.

It may seem surprising that the first medical school should have arisen in the southern part of Italy, but for those who know the historical conditions it will seem the most natural thing in the world that this development should have come in this region. As we have said, touch with Greek has always been the most important factor for modern educational and intellectual development. Salerno was situated in the heart of that Greek colony in the southern part of Italy which came to be known as Magna Græcia. Apparently at no time during the Middle

Ages was Greek entirely a dead language in this part of Italy, and there were Greek travellers, Greek sailors, and many other wanderers, who made their way along the shores of the Mediterranean at this time, and carried with them everywhere the stimulus that always came from association with the Greeks of Asia Minor and of the Grecian Islands and peninsula.

There were two other factors that made for the development of the medical school at Salerno. The first of these seems undoubtedly to have been the presence of the Benedictines, who had a rather important school at Salerno, and who were closely in touch with their great mother-house at Monte Cassino not far away. It was they who imparted the academic atmosphere to the town, and made it possible to gather together the elements for the university which gradually came into existence around the medical school, after that began to attract European attention.

The actual foundation of the medical school, however, seems to have been due to the fortunate accident that Salerno became a health resort, a place to which invalids were attracted from many parts of Europe because the climate was salubrious, and opportunities for obtaining the medical advice of men of many different schools of thought from all over the Mediterranean, and securing the Oriental drugs which were so much valued—as drugs from a distance always are—were there afforded. It is easy to understand that, especially in the winter-time, better-class patients from all over Europe would be glad to go down to the mild temperate climate of Salerno and spend their time there.

It has been pointed out that the first modern university, that of Salerno, had for a nucleus a medical school, representing man's interest in his body as his primary intellectual purpose in modern history. The second modern university, that of Bologna, gathered around a law school representing man's interest in his property—his second formal purpose in life. And the third, that of Paris, developed around a school of theology and philosophy, demonstrating that man's intellectual interests rise finally to the consideration of his relations to his fellow-man and to God.

The first that we know definitely about the medical school of Salerno, the origin of which is difficult to trace, is concerned with Alphanus, usually designated "the First," because there are several of the name. He was a Benedictine monk, distinguished as a literary man and known by his contemporaries as both poet and physician, who was afterwards raised to the Bishopric of Salerno. He had taught at Salerno in the Benedictine school there before becoming Bishop, and when exercising the highest ecclesiastical authority did much to encourage the development of Salerno. He states that medicine flourished in the town even in the ninth century, and there is an old chronicle published by De Renzi in his "Collectio Salernitana" in which it is said that the medical school was founded by four doctors—a Jewish Rabbi, Elinus; a Greek, Pontus; a Saracen, Adale; and the fourth a native of Salerno—each of whom lectured in his native language. This reads like a mythical legend that has formed around some real tradition of the coming of physicians from many countries. Puschmann in his "History of Medical Education" has suggested that the names are probably as much varied as the absolute truth of the facts. Elinus, the Jew, is probably Elias or Eliseus, Adale is probably a corruption of Abdallah, and Pontus should be probably Gariopontus.

There was a hospital at Salerno that was somewhat famous as early as the first quarter of the ninth century. This was placed under the control of the Benedictines; and other infirmaries and charitable institutions, similarly under the care of religious orders, sprang up in Salerno to accommodate the patients that came. The practical character of the teaching at Salerno, as preserved for us in the writings of the school, would seem to argue that probably those who came to study medicine here were brought directly in contact with the patients, though we have no definite evidence of that fact.

The most interesting feature of the medical school at Salerno is undoubtedly the development of legal standards of medical education in connection with the school. Before the middle of the twelfth century Roger, King of the Two Sicilies, issued a decree according to which preliminary studies at the University were required as a preparation for the medical school, and four years of medical studies were made the minimum requirement for the degree of doctor in medicine, which was, however, as we have said, not a licence to practise, but only a certificate authorizing teaching. There seemed to have been, even thus early, some further state regulations with regard to practice. About the middle of the next century, however, there came, through a law of the Emperor Frederick II., a still further evolution of legal standards for medical education and medical practice in the Two Sicilies. This law required that the student of medicine should have spent some years, probably the equivalent of our undergraduate training, in the university before studying medicine, and that he should then devote four years to medicine, after which, on proper examination, he might be given the degree of doctor—that is, teacher of medicine; but he must spend a further year of practice with a physician before he would be allowed to practise for himself.

This is such a high standard that, only that we have the actual wording of the law, it would seem almost impossible that it could have been evolved at this period in medical history. It actually represents the standard that we have climbed back to generally only during the past generation or two, and in the interval there have been many rather serious derogations from it. This law of the Emperor Frederick is, moreover, a pure drug law, regulating the sale of drugs and their purity, and inflicting condign punishment for substitution; in this regard also anticipating our most recent well-considered legislation. The penalty by which the druggist was fined all his movable goods for substitution, while the government inspector who permitted such substitution was put to death, would seem to us in the modern time to make the punishment eminently fit the crime. Almost needless to say, then, the law (see Appendix for full text) represents one of the most important documents in the history of medicine, particularly of medical education. The fee regulation included in it shows that medicine was looked upon as a profession, and was paid accordingly.

From Salerno come many of the traditions of the conferring of degrees which are still used in a large number of modern medical schools. Before receiving his degree, the candidate had to take an oath, of which the following were the principal tenets: "Not to contradict the teaching of his college, not to teach what was false or lying, and not to receive fees from the poor even though they were offered; to commend the sacrament of penance to his patients, to make no dishonest agreement with the druggists, to administer no abortifacient drug to the pregnant, and to prescribe no medicament that was poisonous to human bodies."

It has sometimes been said that youths of tender age were admitted to the study of medicine at Salerno, and that many of them were given their degrees at the age of twenty-one. De Renzi's discussion would seem to show that the usual age of receiving the degree was twenty-five to twenty-seven. As medical students had to have three years of preparatory studies in literature and philosophy, it would seem that they must have been rather mature on their admission to the medical schools.

De Renzi tells us that the medical school of Salerno was of great importance not only for medical education, but it acquired sufficient means to extend its benefits over the entire city. Gifts were made of statues to the churches, and especially to the shrine of St. Matthew the Apostle, situated here; monuments were set up, inscriptions placed and ample donations made to the various institutions of the city. The formal name of the medical school was *Almum et Hippocraticum Medicorum Collegium*. This is the first use that I know of the word *almum* in connection with a college, and may very well be the distant source of our term *alma mater*. The medical school was situated in the midst of an elevated valley which opened up on the mountain that dominates Salerno, and while enjoying very pure air must have been scarcely disturbed at all by the winds which can be blustery enough from the gulf. De Renzi says that in his time some of the remains could still be seen, though visitors to Salerno now come away very much disappointed because nothing of interest is left.

The most famous of the teachers at Salerno was Constantine Africanus, so called because he was born near Carthage. His life runs from the early part of the eleventh century to near its close, and he lived probably well beyond eighty years of age. Having studied medicine in his native town, he wandered through the East, became familiar with a number of Oriental languages, and studied the Arabian literature of science, and above all of medicine, very diligently. The Arabs, owing to their intimate contact with the Greeks in Asia Minor, had the Greek authors constantly before them, and Hippocrates and Galen have always roused men to do good work in medicine. Constantine seems not to have learned Greek, finding enough to satisfy him in the Arabic commentaries on the Greek authors, and probably confident, as all young men have ever been, that what his own time was doing must represent an advance over the Greek. He brought back with him Arabian books and a thorough knowledge of Arabian medicine. When he settled down in Carthage he was accused of magical practices, his medical colleagues being apparently jealous of his success—at least, there is a tradition to that effect to account for his removal to Salerno, though the immediate reason seems to have been that his reputation attracted the attention of Duke Robert of Salerno, who invited him to become his physician.

After Constantine's time the principal textbooks of the school became, according to De Renzi, Hippocrates, Galen, and Avicenna. To these were added the *Antidotarium* of Mesue, and there were various compendiums of medical knowledge, quite as in our own time—one well known under the name of *Articella*. In surgery the principal textbook was the surgical works of the Four Masters of Salerno, which interestingly enough was the sort of combination work gathered from a series of masters that we are accustomed to see so frequently at the present day. De Renzi insists that there was much less Arabic influence at Salerno than is usually thought; and Gurlt more recently has emphasized, as we have said, the fact that the great textbooks of surgery which we have from Salerno contain not Arabisms, as might be expected from the traditions of Arabic influence that we hear so much of, but Græcisms, which show that here at Salerno there was a very early Renaissance, and the influence of Greek writers was felt even in the twelfth century.

Probably the best way to convey in brief form a good idea of the teaching in medicine at Salerno is to quote the *Regimen Sanitatis Salernitanum*, the Code of Health of the School of Salernum, which for many centuries was popular in Europe, and was issued in many editions even after the invention of printing. Professor Ordronaux, Professor of Medical Jurisprudence in the law school of Columbia College (now Columbia University, New York), issued a translation of it in verse,[3] which gives a very good notion of the contents and the spirit and the mode of expression of the little volume.

The *Regimen* was written in the rhymed verses which were so familiar at this time. Many writers on the history of medicine have marvelled at this use of verse, but anyone who knows how many verse-makers there were in the twelfth and thirteenth centuries all over Europe will not be surprised. It used to be the custom to make little of these rhymed Latin verses of the Middle Ages, but it may be well to recall that in recent years a great change has come over the appreciation of the world of literature in their regard. The rhymed Latin hymns of the Church, especially the *Dies Iræ*, the *Stabat Mater*, and others, are now looked upon as representing some of the greatest poetry that ever was written. Professor Saintsbury of the University of Edinburgh has declared them the most wondrous wedding of sense and sound that the world has ever known. The *Regimen Sanitatis* of Salerno is of course no such poetry, mainly because its subject was commonplace and it could not rise to poetic heights. A good deal of the deprecation of its Latinity might well be spared, for most of the mistakes are undoubtedly due to copyists and interpolation. The verses not only rhyme at the end, but often there are internal sub-rhymes. This too was a very common custom among the hymn-writers, as the great sequence of Bernard of Morlaix, so well known through its translations in our time, as "Jerusalem the Golden" attests. The *Regimen* was not written for physicians, but for popular information. It seems to have been a compilation of maxims of health from various professors of the Salernitan School. Nothing that I know shows more clearly the genuine knowledge of medicine, and the careful following of the first rule of medical practice *non nocere* to which Salerno had reached at this time, than the fact that this popular volume contained no recommendation of specific remedies, but only health rules for diet, air, exercise, and the like, many of which are as valuable in our time as they were in that, and very few of which have been entirely superseded—together with some general information as to simples, and a few details of medical knowledge that would give a convincing air to the compilation. The book was dedicated to the King of the English, *Anglorum regi scribit schola tota Salerni*, and in the translation made by Professor Ordonaux begins as follows:

If thou to health and vigour wouldst attain,
 Shun weighty cares—all anger deem profane,
 From heavy suppers and much wine abstain.
 Nor trivial count it, after pompous fare,
 To rise from table and to take the air.

Shun idle, noonday slumber, nor delay
The urgent calls of Nature to obey.
These rules if thou wilt follow to the end,
Thy life to greater length thou mayst extend.[4]

Evidently it was rather easy to commit such rhymes to memory, and this accounts for the fact that we have many different versions of the *Regimen* and disputed readings of all kinds. These medieval hygienists believed very much in early rising, cold water, thorough cleansing, exercise in the open air, yet without sudden cooling afterwards. The lines on morning hygiene seem worth while giving in Ordonaux's translation.

At early dawn, when first from bed you rise,
Wash, in cold water, both your hands and eyes.
With brush and comb then cleanse your teeth and hair,
And thus refreshed, your limbs outstretch with care.
Such things restore the weary, o'ertasked brain;
And to all parts ensure a wholesome gain.
Fresh from the bath, get warm. Rest after food,
Or walk, as seems most suited to your mood.
But in whate'er engaged, or sport, or feat,
Cool not too soon the body when in heat.

The Salernitan writers were not believers in noonday sleep, though one might have expected that the tradition of the *siesta* in Italy had been already established. They insist that it makes one feel worse rather than better to break the day by a sleep at noonday.

Let noontide sleep be brief, or none at all;
Else stupor, headache, fever, rheums, will fall
On him who yields to noontide's drowsy call.

They believed in light suppers—

Great suppers will the stomach's peace impair;
Wouldst lightly rest, curtail thine evening fare.

With regard to the interval between meals, the Salernitan rule was, wait until your stomach is surely empty:

Eat not again till thou dost certain feel
Thy stomach freed of all its previous meal.
This mayst thou know from hunger's teasing call,
Or mouth that waters—surest sign of all.

Pure air and sunlight were favourite tonics at Salerno—

Let air you breathe be sunny, clear, and light,
 Free from disease or cess-pool's fetted blight.

Taking "a hair of the dog that bit you" was, however, a maxim with Salernitans for the cure of potation headaches.

Art sick from vinous surfeiting at night?
 Repeat the dose at morn, 'twill set thee right.

The tradition with regard to the difficulty of the digestion of pork, which we are trying to combat in the modern time, had already been established at Salerno. The digestibility of pork could, however, be improved by good wine.

Inferior far to lamb is flesh of swine,
 Unqualified by gen'rous draughts of wine;
 But add the wine, and lo! you'll quickly find
 In them both food and medicine combined.

Milk for consumptives was a favourite recommendation. The tradition had come down from very old times, and Galen insisted that fresh air and milk and eggs was the best possible treatment for consumption. The Salernitan physicians recommended various kinds of milk, goat's, camel's, ass's, and sheep's milk as well as cow's. It is probable, as I pointed out in my "Psychotherapy," that the mental influence of taking some one of the unusual forms of milk did a good deal to produce a favourable reaction in consumptives, who are so prone to be affected favourably by unusual remedies. The *Regimen* warned, however, that milk will not be good if it produces headache or if there is fever. Apparently some patients had been seen with the idiosyncrasy for milk, and the tendency to constipation and disturbance after it which have been noted also in the modern time.

Goat's milk and camel's, as by all is known,
 Relieve poor mortals in consumption thrown;
 While ass's milk is deemed far more nutritious,
 And e'en beyond all cow's or sheep's, officious.
 But should a fever in the system riot,
 Or headache, let the patient shun this diet.

Salerno's common sense with regard to diet is very well illustrated by a number of maxims. Diet tinkering was not much in favour.

We hold that men on no account should vary
 Their daily diet until necessary:
 For, as Hippocrates doth truly show,
 Diseases sad from all such changes flow.
 A stated diet, as it is well known,

Of physic is the strongest cornerstone—
By means of which, if you can nought impart,
Relief or cure, vain is your Healing Art.

They believed firmly that many of the conditions of eating were quite as important as the diet itself, and said:

Doctors should thus their patients' food revise—
What is it? *When* the meal? And what its *size*?
How *often*? *Where?* lest, by some sad mistake,
Ill-sorted things should meet and trouble make.

They recommended the various simples, mallow, mint, sage, rue, the violet for headache and catarrh, the nettle, mustard, hyssop, elecampane, pennyroyal, cresses, celandine, saffron, leeks—a sovereign remedy for sterility—pepper, fennel, vervaine, henbane, and others. There were certain special affections, as hoarseness, catarrh, headaches, fistula, for which specific directions for cure were given. Here for instance are the directions to be given a patient suffering from rheum or catarrh. The verses conveyed interesting information with nice long names for the various affections, as well as the directions for its management.

Fast well and watch. Eat hot your daily fare,
Work some, and breathe a warm and humid air;
Of drink be spare; your breath at time suspend;
These things observe if you your cold would end.
A cold whose ill-effects extend as far
As in the chest, is known as a catarrh;
Bronchitis, if into the throat it flows;
Coryza, if it reach alone the nose.

The *Regimen* conveyed a deal of information in compact form. It gives the number of bones in the body as 219 with 32 teeth, and the number of veins as 365, this number being chosen doubtless because of some supposed relation to the number of days in the year. It contains also a good brief account of the four humours in the human body—black bile, blood, phlegm, and yellow bile; and of the four temperaments—the sanguine, the bilious, the phlegmatic, and the melancholy. These four temperaments were discussed at considerable length by all the psychologists and most of the writers on religious life for centuries afterwards, largely on the basis of the information conveyed by the Salernitan handbook. There are descriptions of the symptoms of plethora or excess of blood, of excess of bile, of excess of phlegm, and excess of black bile. The little volume finally contains discussions as to bleeding, its indications, contraindications, as in youth—"Ere seventeen years we scarce need drawing blood"—and in old age; and then of the mode of practising it, and the place whence the blood should be drawn to relieve different symptoms.[5]

Salerno impressed itself much more deeply on surgery than on medicine, for the magnificent development of medieval surgery, the knowledge of which has proved so surprising in our day, began down at Salerno. Some of the details of this phase of Salernitan accomplishment are given in the chapter on Medieval Surgeons of Italy. Roger and Roland and the Four Masters were great original founders in a phase of medical science that proved extremely important for the next three or four centuries. Undoubtedly the presence of a hospital at Salerno, where there were gathered a number of the chronic cases from all over Europe, most of them of the better-to-do classes looking for ease from their ills, gave the incentive to this development. When the natural means of cure, tried for a considerable time, failed, recourse was had to surgery for relief, and often with excellent results. This chapter on Salerno's history shows how thoroughgoing was the effort of the members of the faculty of the medical school to develop every possible means of aid for their patients, even when that required pioneer work.

Pagel's appreciation of Salerno's place in the history of medicine, in his chapter on Medicine in the Middle Ages in Puschmann's "Handbuch Der Geschichte der Medicin," Berlin, 1902, gives in very brief space a summary of what was accomplished at Salerno that emphasizes what has been said here, and his authority will confirm those who might possibly continue to doubt of any institution of the Middle Ages having achieved so much. He said:

"If we take up now the accomplishments of the School of Salerno in the different departments, there is one thing that is very remarkable. It is the rich, independent productivity with which Salerno advanced the banners of medical science for hundreds of years, almost as the only autochthonous centre of medical influence in the whole West. One might almost say that it was like a *versprengten Keim*—a displaced embryonic element—which, as it unfolded, rescued from destruction the ruined remains of Greek and Roman medicine. This productivity of Salerno, which may well be compared in quality and quantity with that of the best periods of our science, and in which no department of medicine was left without some advance, is one of the striking phenomena of the history of medicine. While positive progress was not made, there are many noteworthy original observations to be chronicled. It must be acknowledged that pupils and scholars set themselves faithfully to their tasks to further, as far as their strength allowed, the science and art of healing. In the medical writers of the older period of Salerno, who had not yet been disturbed by Arabian culture or scholasticism, we cannot but admire the clear, charmingly smooth, easy-flowing diction, the delicate and honest setting forth of cases, the simplicity of their method of treatment, which was to a great extent dietetic and expectant; and while we admire the carefulness and yet the copiousness of their therapy, we cannot but envy them a certain austerity in their pharmaceutic formulas, and an avoidance of medicamental polypragmasia. The work in internal medicine was especially developed. The contributions to it from a theoretic and literary standpoint, as well as from practical applications, came from ardent devotees."

One very interesting contribution to medical literature that comes to us from Salerno bears the title "The Coming of a Physician to His Patient, or an Instruction for the Physician Himself." It illustrates very well the practical nature of the teaching of Salerno, and gives a rather vivid picture of the medical customs of the time. The instruction as to the conduct of the physician when he first comes into the house and is brought to the patient runs as follows:

"When the doctor enters the dwelling of his patient, he should not appear haughty, nor covetous, but should greet with kindly, modest demeanour those who are present, and then seating himself near the sick man accept the drink which is offered him [*sic*], and praise in a few words the beauty of the neighbourhood, the situation of the house, and the well-known generosity of the family—if it should seem to him suitable to do so. The patient should be put at his ease before the examination begins, and the pulse should be felt deliberately and carefully. The fingers should be kept on the pulse at least until the hundredth beat in order to judge of its kind and character; the friends standing round will be all the more impressed because of the delay, and the physician's words will be received with just that much more attention."

The rest of the advice smacks rather more of sophistication than we care to think of in a professional man, but its display of a profound knowledge of human nature makes it interesting.

"On the way to see the sick person he (the physician) should question the messenger who has summoned him upon the circumstances and the conditions of the illness of the patient; then, if not able to make any positive diagnosis after examining the pulse and the urine, he will at least excite the patient's astonishment by his accurate knowledge of the symptoms of the disease, and thus win his confidence."

Salerno taught as well as it could the science of medicine, and initiated great advances in surgery; but it also emphasized the art of medicine, and recognized very clearly that the personality of the physician counted for a great deal, and that his influence upon his patients must be fostered quite as sedulously as his knowledge of the resources of medicine for their ills.

CHAPTER IV

MONTPELLIER AND MEDICAL EDUCATION IN THE WEST

After Salerno the next great medical school was that of Montpellier in the South of France. The conditions which brought about its original establishment are very like those which occasioned the foundation of Salerno. Montpellier, situated not far from the Mediterranean, came to be a health resort. Patients flocked to it from many countries of the West of Europe; physicians settled there because patients were numerous, and medical instruction came to be offered to students. Fame came to the school. The fundamental reason for this striking development of the intellectual life seems to have been that Montpellier was not far from Marseilles, which had been a Greek colony originally and continued to be under Greek influence for many centuries. As a consequence of this the artistic and intellectual life of the southern part of France was higher during the earlier Middle Ages than that of any other part of Europe, except certain portions of South Italy. The remains of the magnificent architecture of the Roman period are well known, and Provence has always been famous for its intellectual and literary life. Among a people who were in this environment, we might well look for an early renaissance of education.

It is not surprising, then, that one of the earliest of the medical schools of modern history around which there gradually developed a university should have come into existence in this part of the world. What is even more interesting perhaps for us, is that this medical school has persisted down to our own day, and has always been, for nearly ten centuries now, a centre of excellent medical education.

There gathered around the story of its origin such legends as were noted with regard to the history of Salerno, and there is no doubt that Jewish and Moorish physicians who became professors there contributed not a little to the prestige of the school and the reputation that it acquired throughout Europe. The attempt to attribute all of the stimulus for the intellectual life at Montpellier to these foreign elements is, however, simply due to that paradoxical state of mind which has so often tried to minimize the value of Christian contributions to science and the intellectual life, even by the exaggeration of the significance of what came from foreign and un-Christian sources. Proper recognition must be accorded to both Jewish and Moorish factors at Montpellier, but the one important element is that these foreign professors brought with them, even though always in rather far-fetched translations, the ideas of the great Greek masters of medicine to which the region and the people around Montpellier were particularly sensitive, because of the Greek elements in the population, and hence the development of a significant centre of education here.

The date of the rise of the medical school at Montpellier is, as suggested by Puschmann, veiled in the obscurity of tradition. There seems to be no doubt that it goes back to as early as the tenth century, it was already famous in the eleventh, and it attracted students from all over Europe during the twelfth century. When Bishop Adalbert of Mainz came thither in 1137, the school possessed buildings of its own, as we learn from the words of a contemporary, Bishop Anselm of Havelberg. St. Bernard in a letter written in 1153 tells that the Archbishop of Lyons, being ill, repaired to Montpellier to be under the treatment of the physicians there. Perhaps the most interesting feature of this letter is the fact that the good Archbishop not only spent what money he had with him on physicians, but ran into debt.

The two schools, Salerno and Montpellier, came to be mentioned by writers of the period as representing the twins of medical learning of the time. John of Salisbury, a writer of the early thirteenth century, declares that those who wished to devote themselves to medicine at this time went either to Salerno or Montpellier. Ægidius or Gilles de Corbeil, the well-known physician, and Hartmann von der Aue, the Meistersinger, both mention Salerno and Montpellier, usually in association, in their writings, and make it very clear that in the West at least the two names had come to be almost invariably connected as representing rival medical schools of about equal prominence.

The reputation of Montpellier spread in Italy also, however, and we have the best evidence for this from an incident that took place in Rome at the beginning of the thirteenth century, which is more fully dwelt on in the chapter on Medieval Hospitals. Pope Innocent III. wanted to create a model hospital at Rome, and made inquiries as to who would be best fitted to organize such an institution. He was told of the work of Guy or Guido of Montpellier, who was a member of the Order of the Holy Ghost and had made a great hospital at Montpellier. Accordingly Guy was summoned to Rome, and the establishment of the Santo Spirito Hospital was entrusted to him. It was on the model of this that a great many hospitals were founded throughout the world, for Pope Innocent insisted that every diocese in Christianity should have a hospital, and Bishops who came on formal visits to the Holy See were asked to inspect the Santo Spirito for guidance in their own diocesan hospital establishments. Many of the hospitals throughout the world came as a result to be hospitals of the Holy Ghost and this contribution alone of Montpellier to the medical world of the time was of great significance and must have added much to her prestige.

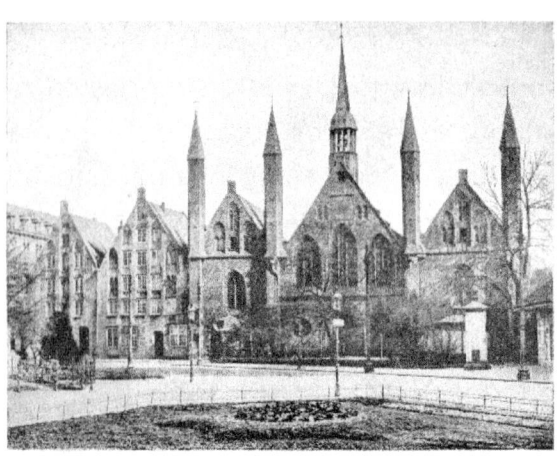

HOLY GHOST HOSPITAL (LÜBECK)
From "The Thirteenth: Greatest of Centuries," by J. J. Walsh

Montpellier, like Salerno, seems to have attracted students to its medical school from all over the world. There were undoubtedly many English there, and probably also Irish and Scotch, though the journey must have been much longer and more difficult to make than is that from America to Europe at the present time. Of course there came many from Spain and from North France and the Netherlands. The fact that a number of Italians went there before the close of the Middle Ages shows how deeply interested were the men of this time in knowledge for its own sake, and indicates that something of that internationality of culture which we are priding ourselves on at the present time, because our students from all countries go far afield for postgraduate work and there is an interchange of professors, existed at this period. In spite of the fact that books were only written by hand, the teaching of distinguished professors had a wide diffusion, and students were quite ready to go through the drudgery of making these handwritten copies of a favourite master's work. They had plenty of common sense as well as powers of observation, and some of their writing is still of great practical value.

A number of men who are famous in the history of medicine made their medical studies at Montpellier in the twelfth and thirteenth centuries. Among them are Mondeville, who afterwards taught surgery at Paris; and Guy de Chauliac, who was a Papal Physician at Avignon and at the same time a professor at Montpellier, probably spending a certain number of weeks, or perhaps months, each year in the university town. Sketches of these men, and of other students and teachers at Montpellier who reached distinction in surgery, will be found in the chapter on Surgeons of the West of Europe. Some other distinguished Montpellierians deserve brief mention.

One of the distinguished professors at Montpellier was the well-known Arnold de Villanova, of whose name there are a number of variants, including even Rainaldus and Reginaldus. In 1285 he was already a famous physician, and was sent for to treat Peter III., King of Aragon, who was severely ill. In 1299 he was summoned on a consultation to the bedside of King Philip the Handsome (le Bel) at Paris. After this we hear of him in many places, as at the Court of Pope Benedict XI. at Rome, and in 1308 as the physician and friend of Pope Clement V. at Avignon. His writings were printed in a number of editions in the Renaissance time, Venice 1505, Lyons 1509, 1520, 1532, Basel 1585, and his medical and astronomical and chemical works in separate volumes at Lyons in 1586.

His aphorisms are well known, and used to be frequently quoted during the Middle Ages and afterwards, and some of them deserve to be remembered even at the present time. For instance, he said: "Where the veins and arteries are notably large, incision and deep cauterization should be avoided." "When cauterization is to be done the direct cautery should be used; caustic applications are only suitable for very timid patients." "The lips of a wound will glue together of themselves if there is no foreign substance between them, and in this way the natural appearance of the part will be preserved." "In large wounds sutures should be used, and silk thread tied at short distances makes the best sutures." "The infection of the dura mater is followed in most cases by death." "A collection of pus is best dissolved by incision and cleaning out of the purulent material." "To put off the opening of an abscess brings many dangers with it." "In most cases of scrofula external applications are better than the use of the knife. Scrofulous patients always have other sources of infection within them, and so it does them no good to operate externally." "Tranquil and pure air is the best friend for convalescents."

Villanova advised that the bite of a mad dog should not be permitted to heal at once, but the wound should be enlarged and allowed to bleed freely, leeches and cups being used to encourage bleeding, and healing should not be permitted for forty days. He believed very thoroughly in drainage, and in the dilation of narrow fistulous openings. He describes anthrax or carbuncle, and has chapters on various painful conditions for which he employs the terms arthritis, sciatica, chiragra, podagra, and gonagra.

Villanova's treatment of the subject of hernia shows how thoroughly conservative he was, and how careful were his observations. In young persons in recent hernias he advised immediate complete reposition of the contents of the sac, the bringing together of the hernial opening by means of adhesive plaster, above which a bandage was placed, and the patient should be put to bed with the feet and legs elevated and the head depressed for ten to fifteen days or more if necessary. He says that "there are some—especially surgeons—who claim that they can cure hernia by incision, and some others by means of a purse-string ligature, and still others by the cautery or by some cauterizing material [they manifestly had our complete catalogue of 'fakes' in the matter]; but I prefer not to mention these procedures, since I have seen many patients perish under them, and others brought into serious danger of death, and I do not think that the surgeon will acquire glory or an increase of his friends from such perilous procedures, and I do not approve their use."

One of the important writers of Montpellier was Gilbertus Anglicus (Gilbert the Englishman), who is called in one of the old translations of Mesue Doctor *Desideratissimus*, which I suppose might be Anglicized "loveliest of doctors." After his studies in England he went for graduate work to some of the famous foreign universities, and is named as a chancellor of Montpellier. His best-known work is his "Compendium Medicinæ," which bore as its full title "The Compendium of Medicine of Gilbert the Englishman; useful not only to physicians, but to clergymen for the treatment of all and every disease." Gurlt says that it contains little that is original, being a copy of Roger of Parma and Theodoric of Lucca, with a number of quotations from the Arabs, nearly all of whom Gilbert seems to have read with considerable attention. It is interesting to find that Gilbert was definitely of the opinion that cancer is incurable except by incision or cauterization. He declares that it yields to no medicine except surgery.

Another of the men whose names are connected with Montpellier was John of Gaddesden, often called *Joannes Anglicus*. He was a student of Merton College, and received his degree of doctor of medicine at Oxford. He studied afterwards at Montpellier and also at Paris, and settled down to practise in London. He treated the son of King Edward II. for smallpox, and having wrapped him in red cloth and made all the hangings of his bed red, so that the patient was completely surrounded by this colour, he declared that he made "a good cure, and I cured him without any vestiges of the pocks." The treatment is interesting, as an anticipation in a certain way of Finsen's red light treatment for smallpox in our own time. Hanging the room, and especially the doors and the windows, with red when smallpox was to be treated was a favourite treatment down at Montpellier. Gaddesden's book is called by the somewhat fanciful name "Rosa Anglica." Bernard Gordon of Montpellier had written a "Lilium Medicinæ," and we have a "Flos Medicinæ" from Salerno, so that flower names for medical textbooks were evidently the fashion of the time.

Gaddesden's book is almost entirely a compilation, and except in the relation of his surgical experience, contains little that is new. Guy de Chauliac was quite impatient with it, and declared that "lately there had arisen a foolish Anglican rose which was sent to me and I looked it over. I expected to find the odour of sweetness in it, but I found only some old fables." The criticism is, however, as Gurlt remarks, too severe and not quite justified, representing rather Guy's high ideal of the originality that a new textbook should possess, than a legitimate critical opinion. If our own textbooks were to be judged by any such lofty standard, most of them would suffer rather severely.

Another of the well-known teachers at Montpellier was Valesco de Taranta. There are the usual variants of his name, his first name being written also Balesco, and his last name sometimes Tharanta. He was a Portuguese who studied in Lisbon, and later in Montpellier, where he taught afterwards and was considered one of the distinguished professors of his day, being for a time chancellor. He became so well known that he was summoned in consultation to the French King Charles VI., and there is some doubt as to whether he did not become his regular physician. One of his works, the "Philonium Pharmaceuticum et Chirurgicum de medendis omnibus, cum internis tum externis, humani corporis affectionibus," had the honour of being printed at Lyons in two editions in 1490, and one at Venice the same year, at Lyons 1500, Venice 1502, Lyons 1516, 1521, 1532, 1535, Venice 1589, and Lyons 1599. It has also been reprinted subsequently in a number of editions, so that it must have been a much-read book. Valesco had two favourite authors, Galen and Guy de Chauliac. The fact that he should have appreciated two such great men so thoroughly is of itself the best evidence of his own ability and critical judgment. His book, from the number of printed editions, must have been in the hands of practically all the progressive physicians of the southern part of France, at least during the fifteenth, sixteenth, and part of the seventeenth centuries.

A very well-known teacher of Montpellier, who has had a reputation in English-speaking countries because his name was supposed to indicate that he was a Scotchman, was Bernard Gordon or de Gordon, whose name is, however, also written Gourdon. He was a teacher at Montpellier at the end of the thirteenth and the beginning of the fourteenth century. His textbook of medicine, in accordance with the custom of the time, is called by the flowery title "Lilium Medicinæ," the Lily of Medicine. While much of his information was derived from the Arabs, some of his teaching was an advance on theirs, and he described the acute fevers, leprosy, scabies, anthrax, as well as erysipelas, and still more strangely phthisis, as contagious. Dr. Garrison has called attention in his "History of Medicine" to the fact that the book is notable as containing the first description of a modern truss, and a very early mention of spectacles under the Latin name *oculus berellinus*. In recent years it has come to be the custom to think of Gordon or Gourdon as probably not of Scotch but of French origin—that is, born somewhere in the confines of what we now call France. There are a number of French places of the name of Gourdon from any of which he might have come.

Montpellier represented for the West of Europe then very nearly what Salerno did for Italy and Eastern Europe. It very probably attracted many of the English and Scotch students of medicine, though not all the names supposed to be of British origin have proved to be so with the development of our knowledge. Montpellier has survived, however, while Salerno disappeared as a force in medical education. Its story would well deserve telling in detail, and doubtless the new national spirit of the French after the war will prove an incentive to the writing of it.

CHAPTER V

LATER MEDIEVAL MEDICINE

Medicine in the later Middle Ages, that is, from the tenth to the middle of the fifteenth centuries, was greatly influenced by the medical schools which arose in Italy and the West of Europe during this period. These were organized mainly in connection with universities, Salerno, Montpellier, Bologna, Paris, Padua, in the order of their foundations, so far as they can be ascertained. These university medical schools represented serious scientific teaching in medicine, and certainly were not more prone to accept absurdities of therapeutics and other phases of supposed medical knowledge than have been the universities of any other corresponding period of time. Five centuries represent a very long interval in the history of humanity, and provide opportunities for a great many curious developments and ups and downs of interest, all of which must not be considered as representing any particular generation or even century in the history of that time. The absurdities came and went quite as in more modern times; but all the while there was an undercurrent of solid medical knowledge, founded on observation and definite clinical research, superadded to the information obtained from the classics of medicine.

Even as early as the tenth century the thoroughly conservative teaching of Salerno in medicine made itself felt, and above all counteracted the Oriental tendencies to over-refinement of drugging, which had led to the so-called calendar prescription. This was the most noteworthy element in the medical practice of the later Middle Ages, but its significance has been dwelt on in the chapter on Salerno and the Beginnings of Medical History. While Arabic polypharmacy is the most striking feature of Mohammedan influence on medicine at this time, there were a number of Arabian and Jewish physicians who made a deep impression on the medicine of the later Middle Ages—that is, subsequent to the tenth century. Their work was felt not only in their own time, but for many subsequent centuries even down to and beyond the Renaissance, and they therefore must find a place in medieval medical history. This influence was exerted ever so much more outside of Italy than in the Italian peninsula, where the tradition of their contact with the original Greek authors still remained, and where they were making medicine and surgery for themselves quite apart from Arabian influence.

The more one knows about the conditions in Italian medicine the less question is there of Arabian contributions to it. De Renzi in his History of Italian Medicine makes it very clear that the Arabs exercised no significant influence either at

Salerno or elsewhere. The Benedictines and Cassiodorus afford evidence of the study of the Greek medical classics in Latin translations. Muratori cites a manuscript which he had consulted in the Medicean Library at Florence, and which, though written between the eighth and ninth centuries, says not a word of the Arabs and bears the title of "Abstracts from Hippocrates, Galen, Oribasius, Heliodorus, Asclepiades, Archigenes, Dioclis, Amyntas, Apollonius, Nymphiodorus, Ruffius, Ephesinus, Soranus, Ægineta, and Palladius." These and not the Arabs were the masters of the Italians, and it was fortunate, for the world was thus saved many Arabian mistakes and their tendency to neglect surgery. Before Salerno began to exert its real influence, some of the Arabian physicians came to occupy places of prominence in the medicine of the time.

The most important of these was Avicenna, born toward the end of the tenth century in the Persian province of Chorasan, at the height of Arabian influence. He is sometimes spoken of as the Arabian Galen. His famous book, "The Canon," was the most consulted medical book throughout Europe for centuries. There are very few subjects in medicine that did not receive suggestive treatment at his hands. He has definite information with regard to Bubonic plague and the *filaria medinensis*. He has special chapters with regard to obesity, emaciation, and general constitutional conditions. He has chapters on cosmetics and on affections of the hair and nails that are interesting reading. The Renaissance scholars wrote many commentaries on his work, and for long after the introduction of printing his influence was felt widely.

His Arabic colleague in the West was Avenzoar, to call him by the transformation of his Arabic family name, Ibn-Zohr. He was born near Seville, and probably died there, in 1162, well past ninety years of age. He was the teacher of Averröes, who always speaks of him with great respect. He is interesting as probably the first to suggest nutrition per rectum. His apparatus for the purpose consisted of the bladder of a goat with a silver cannula fastened into its neck. Having first carefully washed out the rectum with cleansing and purifying clysters, he injected the nutriment—eggs, milk, and gruel—into the gut. His idea was that the intestine would take this and, as he said, suck it up, carrying it back to the stomach, where it would be digested.

The bladders of animals were very commonly used by these Moorish physicians and by their disciples, and the profession generally, for generations, for a great many purposes for which we now use rubber bags. Abulcasis, for instance, used a sheep's bladder introduced into the vagina and filled with air as a colpeurynter for supporting the organs in the neighbourhood, and also in fractures of the pubic arch.

Avenzoar suggested feeding *per rectum* in cases of stricture of the œsophagus, but he also treated the œsophageal stricture directly. He inserted a cannula of silver through the mouth until its head met an obstruction. This was pushed firmly, but withdrawn whenever there was a vomiting movement, until it became engaged in the stricture. Through it then *freshly milked* milk, or gruel made from farina or barley, was to be poured. He had evidently seen cases improve this way, and therefore must have had experience with functional stricture of the œsophagus. He adds that some physicians believe that nutrition may be absorbed through the pores of the whole body, and that therefore in these cases the patient might be put in a warm milk or gruel bath; but he has not very much faith in the procedure, and says that the reasons urged for it are weak and rather frivolous. It is easy to understand that a man who could recommend manipulative modes of treatment of such kinds, and discuss questions of nutrition so sensibly, knew his medicine very practically and wrote of it judiciously.

Maimonides (1135-1204) was one of these wise old Jews who quotes with approval from a Rabbi of old who had counselled his students: "Teach thy tongue to say, I do not know." Knowing thus the limitations of his own knowledge, it is not surprising that Maimonides should have left a series of practical observations for the maintenance of health which represent the common sense of all time in the matter. Maimonides anticipated the modern rule for taking fruits before meals, as we all do now at breakfast, and so often as fruit cocktails at the beginning of other meals. He thought that grapes, figs, melons, should be taken before meals, and not mixed with other food. He set down as a rule that what was easily digestible should be eaten at the beginning of the meal, to be followed by what was more difficult of digestion. He declared it to be an axiom of medicine "that so long as a man is able to be active and vigorous, does not eat until he is over full, and does not suffer from constipation, he is not liable to disease."

Salerno's influence was felt much more deeply on surgery than on medicine, as can be seen very clearly from the chapter on Medieval Surgeons—Italy. These great surgeons of the period were also the leaders in medicine—for almost needless to say, there was no separation between the two modes of practice—men were as a rule both physicians and surgeons, even though for us their most important work by far was done in surgery. Certain passages from the works of these great surgeons that have come down to us deserve a place in the treatment of the more distinctly medical questions of the time.

Lanfranc the great French surgeon's description of the treatment of the bite of a rabid dog is interesting. He suggests that a large cupping-glass should be applied over the wound, so as to draw out as much blood as possible. After this the wound should be dilated and thoroughly cauterized to its depths with a hot iron. It should then be covered with various substances that were supposed "to draw," in order as far as possible to remove the poison. His description of how one may recognize a rabid animal is rather striking in the light of our present knowledge, for he seems to have realized that the main diagnostic element is a change in the disposition of the animal, but above all a definite tendency to lack playfulness. Lanfranc had manifestly seen a number of cases of true rabies, and describes and suggests treatment for them, though evidently without very much confidence in the success of the treatment.

The treatment of snake-bites and the bites of other animals supposed to be poisonous, or at least suspicious, followed the principles laid down for handling the bite of a mad dog. This was the case particularly as to the encouragement of free bleeding and the use of the cautery.

A characteristic example of the power of clinical observation of the medieval physicians, and one which illustrates much better than many of the absurd tales told as typical of their superstitious tendencies, but really representing that tendency always present in mankind to believe wonders, is to be found in how much they learned of rabies. Even in our own time there are many absurd beliefs with regard to this disease, with some denials of its existence and many grossly exaggerated tales, widely believed; yet the medieval people seem to have reached some quite rational notions with regard to it. Bartholomæus Anglicus is the author of a popular encyclopedia which was very widely read in the medieval period. He was an English Franciscan of the thirteenth century, who gathered together a lot of information and wrote a volume that for centuries after his time, even down to Shakespeare's boyhood, was popular in England.

Here is his description of rabies as he knew it. The most important element is his recognition of the uncertainty of the length of the incubation period, but it contains two other ideas that are very interesting, because medicine in subsequent centuries has come back to them over and over again. One is that free bleeding may remove the virus, and the other that the cautery may help in preventing the infection.

"The biting of a wood-hound is deadly and venomous, and such venom is perilous. For it is long hidden and unknown, and increaseth and multiplieth itself, and is sometimes unknown to the year's end, and then the same day and hour of the biting it cometh to the head, and breedeth frenzy. They that are bitten of a wood-hound have in their sleep dreadful sights, and are fearful, astonished, and wroth without cause. And they dread to be seen of other men, and bark as hounds, and they dread water most of all things, and are afeared thereof, full sore and squeamous also. Against the biting of a wood-hound wise men and ready use to make the wounds bleed with fire or with iron, that the venom may come out with the blood that cometh out of the wound."

A very interesting development of therapeutics in the Middle Ages was the employment of the red light treatment to shorten the course and the severity of the fever in smallpox, and above all to prevent pitting; it was employed successfully by John of Gaddesden in the case of the son of King Edward II. Recent investigation by Cholmeley has shown that both Gilbertus Anglicus (1290) and Bernard de Gordon (1305) antedated John of Gaddesden in references to the red light treatment. All of these men were professors at Montpellier, showing that the medical school of the South of France was a rival in the use of natural methods of cure to its better-known predecessor of Southern Italy. Curiously enough, the "Rosa Anglica" of Gaddesden, in which the reference to the red light is made, is deservedly characterized by Garrison as "a farrago of Arabist quackeries and countrified superstitions"; it well deserves Guy de Chauliac's bitter criticism of it as "a scentless rose."

The idea included under the word autointoxication in our time—that is, that the human body has a tendency to produce poisons within itself, which act deleteriously on it and must be eliminated—was a favourite one during the Middle Ages. It became the custom in our time to have recourse to antiseptics or to surgical measures of various kinds for the relief and prevention of autointoxication. In the Middle Ages they thought to reduce its harmfulness at least by direct elimination, hence the use of drastic purgatives. It seems worth while remarking, however, that the employment of these did not come into general use until the close of the Middle Ages. Basil Valentine, if he really lived in the Middle Ages, and is not merely a name for a writer of the early sixteenth century, as modern historians seem inclined to think, suggested the use of antimony for the removal of the materies morbi from the body that has so much obsessed physicians for many generations. Antimony continued to be used down to the nineteenth century. It was gradually replaced by venesection, which was employed very strenuously during the eighteenth and early nineteenth centuries, in spite of the objection of such men as Morgagni, who refused to allow this mode of treatment to be used on him.

Venesection was succeeded by large doses of calomel, and the calomel era continued on almost to our own generation.

As a rule, however, the medieval physicians trusted nature much more than did their colleagues of modern history—that is, after the Renaissance until the present epoch of medical science began. It has always been difficult, however, for physicians to continue long in the persuasion that nature is a helpful auxiliary, and not a hampering factor to be combated. It is all the more to the credit of the medieval physicians to find, then, that in spite of many absurdities they continued for all the later centuries of the Middle Ages to extol the value of the natural means of cure.

I shall have much to say of John of Ardern in the chapter on Medieval Surgeons of the West of Europe, but he deserves a place also in the chapter on Medicine. Ardern's advice to patients suffering from renal disease, which is contained in a separate tract of his lesser writings with the title in an old English version of "The Governaunce of Nefretykes," is extremely interesting, because it shows very clearly how long ago thoughtful physicians anticipated most of the directions that we now give such patients. Though we are inclined to think that any real knowledge of renal disease is quite modern, and above all has come since Bright's time, this paragraph of Ardern's shows how long before definite pathological knowledge had developed, careful clinical observation worked out empirically the indications of the affection. The paragraph is of special interest, because it contains the first reference to the possible danger that there may be for sufferers from kidney disease using the dark or red meats rather than the white meats. The tradition as to the distinction between the red and white meats has continued ever since his time, and though our modern chemistry does not enable us to find any such distinction between these substances as would justify the differentiation thus dwelt on, it has been maintained for no other reason that I have ever been able to find than because of the long years of tradition and clinical observation behind it.[6]

"Nefretykes must putte awey ire, hyghly and moche besynesse and almanere [business and all manner of] thynge that longeth to the soule saff [save] only joye…. They schulle forbere almanere metys that ben to grete of substaunse and viscous, as olde beeff that is myghtyly pooudryd and enharded with salt and also fressch porke but yf it lye in salt iiii dayes afore…. They mowe use grete wyne and the fflessch of calvys that ben soowkynge and also of all ffowlys saff thoo that ben of the lakys and dichys [dykes?] … and squamous ffyssches, i.e., fyssch of the rivere, of the stony waterys and rennynge ryveres and not of the standyne waterys and they schulle eschywe [eschew] almaner mete made of paast [pastries] and all bred that is dowgh bakene and all fatnesse. And they schulle use the reynes of te beeste other roste or sode. And in especiall he schall use a ffowl that is callyd Cauda tremula or Wagstertte [the wagtail, an English bird] other fressch or salte or bakene withoute drynesse ffor and it be drye it is nought woorth. And note that the use of the powdir or of the flessch of the Wagstertte avayleth gretly to breke the stone in the bladdere."[7]

CHAPTER VI

MEDIEVAL SURGEONS: ITALY

Strange as it may seem, and quite contrary to the usual impressions in the matter, the most interesting department of the history of the medical science during the Middle Ages is that of surgery. Because of this fact we have to divide the subject into two chapters, one for the surgery of Italy, the other for the surgery of the rest of Europe.

We have two series of medieval textbooks which treat largely of surgical subjects in a thoroughly scientific and professional way. The first of these comes to us from the earlier centuries of the Middle Ages, when Greek classic influence on medicine and the medical sciences was on the wane; and the other set comes to us from the later Middle Ages, when the earlier Renaissance of Greek influence was just making itself felt in Europe. Both sets of books serve to show very well that the men of these times were not only deeply interested in the affections for which surgery can provide the only relief possible, but that they had reached very definite, indeed sometimes ultimate, solutions of a large number of the constantly recurring problems of surgery.

The greatest surprise of the whole range of medical history is that these medieval surgeons of both periods anticipated not a few of the surgical advances that we have been accustomed to think of as having been reserved for our time to make. Our knowledge of these details of the work of the medieval surgeons not only of the sixth and seventh centuries, but also of the thirteenth and fourteenth, is not founded on tradition, nor on a few scattered expressions which a modern medievalist might exaggerate, but on actual textbooks, which fortunately for us were reprinted as a rule during the Renaissance period, and have been preserved for us usually in a number of rather readily available copies. Most of them have been reprinted during the past generation, and have revolutionized our knowledge of the history of surgery; for these textbooks exhibit in detail a deep knowledge of surgical affections, a well-developed differential diagnosis, a thoroughly conservative treatment, and yet a distinct effort to give the patient every possible surgical opportunity for his life, compatible with reasonable assurance of successful surgical intervention. As I have pointed out, the surgical history of the old Crusades was as interesting and almost as valuable for civil surgery as that of our own Great War.[8]

Three writers whom we have already mentioned (Early Medieval Medicine)—Aëtius, Alexander of Tralles, and Paul of Ægina—were, as we have seen, all of them interested in surgery, and wrote very interestingly on that subject. It is, however, from the end of the Middle Ages—that is, from the writers of the twelfth century down to the end of the fifteenth—that surprising contributions were made to surgical knowledge. This surgery of the end of the Middle Ages began its development at Salerno. The first great textbook was that of Roger—known also as Rogero and Ruggiero, with the adjective Parmensis or Salernitanus, of Parma or Salerno—who wrote his work about 1180. It is of this that Gurlt, in his "History of Surgery," vol. i., p. 701, says: "Though Arabian works on surgery had been brought over to Italy by Constantine Africanus a hundred years before Roger's time, these exercised no influence over Italian surgery in the next century, and there is scarcely a trace of the surgical knowledge of the Arabs to be found in Roger's works." He insisted, further, that Arabisms are not found in Roger's writings, while many Græcisms occur. The Salernitan School of Surgery drank, then, at the fountain-head of Greek surgery.

After Roger comes Rolando, his pupil, who wrote a commentary on his master's work, and then the combined work of both of them was subsequently annotated by the Four Masters. It is this textbook, the work of many hands and the combined experience of many great teachers, that is the foundation stone of modern surgery. Some of the expressions in this volume will serve to give the best idea of how thoroughly these surgeons of the later medieval period studied their cases, how careful they were in observation, and how well they solved many problems that we are inclined to think of as having come up for serious consideration only much later than this time. After studying their chapter on Injuries of the Head, it is easy to understand why Gurlt should declare that, though there is some doubt about the names of the authors, this volume makes it very clear that these writers drew their opinions from a rich experience.

They warn about the possibility of fracture of the skull even when there is no penetrating wound of the scalp, and they even suggest the advisability of exploratory incision when there is some good reason for suspicion of, though no evident sign of, fracture. In "Old-Time Makers of Medicine," I quoted some of the details of this teaching as to head surgery that may serve to illustrate what these surgeons taught on this important subject.

There are many warnings of the danger of opening the skull, and of the necessity for definitely deciding beforehand that there is good reason for so doing. How carefully their observation had been made, and how well they had taken advantage of their opportunities, which were, of course, very frequent in those warlike times when firearms were unknown, hand-to-hand conflict common, and blunt weapons were often used, can be appreciated very well from some of the directions. For instance, they knew of the possibility of fracture by *contrecoup.*

They say that "quite frequently, though the percussion comes in the anterior part of the cranium, the cranium is fractured on the opposite part." They even seem to have known of accidents such as we now discuss in connection with the laceration of the middle meningeal artery. They warn surgeons of the possibilities of these cases. They tell the story of "a youth who had a very small wound made by a thrown stone, and there seemed no serious results or bad signs. He died the next day, however. His cranium was opened, and a large amount of black blood was found coagulated about his dura mater."

There are many interesting things said with regard to depressed fractures and the necessity for elevating the bone. If the depressed portion is wedged, then an opening should be made with the trephine, and an elevating instrument called a spatumen used to relieve the pressure. Great care should be taken, however, in carrying out this procedure, lest the bone of the cranium itself, in being lifted, should injure the soft structures within. The dura mater should be carefully protected from injury as well as the pia. Care should especially be exercised at the brow, and the rear of the head, and at the commissures (*proram et pupim et commissuras*), since at these points the dura mater is likely to be adherent. Perhaps the most striking expression, the word "infect" being italicized by Gurlt, is: "In elevating the cranium, be solicitous lest you should *infect* or injure the dura mater."

While these old-time surgeons insisted on the necessity for treating all depressed fractures, and even suggested that many fissure fractures required trephining, they deprecated meddlesome surgery of the cranium, unless there was evident necessity, quite as much as we do now. Surgeons who in every serious wound of the head have recourse to the trephine must, they said, be looked upon as fools and idiots (*idioti et stolidi*). When operations were done on the head, cold particularly was to be avoided. The operations were not to be done in cold weather, and above all not in cold places. The air of the operating-room must be warmed artificially. Hot plates should surround the patient's head while the operation was being performed. If this were not possible they were to be done by candlelight, the candle being held as close as possible in a warm room. They had many experiences with fractures at the base of the skull. Hæmorrhages from the mouth and nose and from the ears were considered a bad sign. They even suggested, for diagnostic purposes, what seems to us the rather dangerous procedure that the patient should hold his mouth and nostrils tight shut and blow strongly. One of their methods of negative diagnosis for fractures of the skull was that, if the patient were able to bring his teeth together strongly, or to crack a nut without pain, then there was no fracture present. One of the commentators, however, adds to this, as well he might, *sed hoc aliquando fallit*—"but this sign sometimes fails." Split or crack fractures were also diagnosticated by the methods suggested by Hippocrates of pouring some coloured fluid over the skull after the bone was exposed, when a linear fracture would show by coloration. The Four Masters suggest a sort of red ink for this purpose.

One might well expect that, with trephining as frequent as this textbook of the Four Masters more than hints, the death-rate of these medieval surgeons must have been very high in head cases. We can scarcely understand such intervention in the conditions of operation assumed to exist in the Middle Ages without almost inevitable infection and consequent death. They seem to have come to an empiric recognition of the advantage of absolute cleanliness in such operations. Indeed, in the light of our modern asepsis and its development during our own generation, it is rather startling to note the anticipation of what is most recent in the directions that are given to a surgeon to be observed on the day when he is to do a trephining. I give it in the original Latin as it may be found in Gurlt (vol. i., p. 707): "*Et nota quod die illa cavendum est medico a coitu et malis cibis æra corrumpentibus, ut sunt allia, cepe, et hujusmodi, et colloquio mulieris menstruosæ, et manus ejus debent esse mundæ*, etc." The directions are most interesting. The surgeon's hands must be clean; he must avoid coitus and the taking of food that may corrupt the air, such as onions, leeks, and the like; must avoid menstruating women; and in general must keep himself in a state of absolute cleanliness.

After the South Italian surgeons, some of whom taught at Bologna, a group of North Italian surgeons, most of whom probably were either direct or indirect pupils of the Salernitan School, must be considered. This includes such distinguished names in the history of surgery as Bruno da Longoburgo, usually called simply Bruno; Theodoric and his father Hugh of Lucca; William of Salicet; Lanfranc, the disciple of William who taught at Paris, and gave that primacy to French surgery which was maintained all the centuries down to the nineteenth (p. 1); and Mondino, the author of the first manual on dissection, which continued for two centuries to be used by practically everyone who anywhere did dissection throughout Europe. Practically all of these men did their best work between 1250 and 1300. Bruno of Longoburgo taught at Padua and Vicenza, and his textbook, the "Chirurgia Magna," was completed in Padua in January, 1252. Gurlt notes that "He is the first of the Italian surgeons who besides the Greeks quotes also the Arabian writers on surgery." Eclecticism had definitely come into vogue to replace exclusive devotion to the Greek authors, and men were taking what was good wherever they found it.

Bruno begins his work by a definition of surgery, *chirurgia*, tracing it to the Greek and emphasizing that it means handwork. He then declares that it is the last instrument of medicine to be used, only when the other two instruments, diet and potions, have failed. He insists that surgeons must learn by seeing surgical operations, and watching them long and diligently. They must be neither rash nor over-bold, and should be extremely cautious about operating. While he says that he does not object to a surgeon taking a glass of wine, the followers of this specialty must not drink to such an extent as to disturb their command over themselves, and they must not be habitual drinkers. While all that is necessary for their art cannot be learned out of books, they must not despise books, however, for many things can be learned readily from books, even about the most difficult parts of surgery. Three things the surgeon has to do—"to bring together separated parts, to separate those that have become abnormally united, and to extirpate what is superfluous."

While the old textbooks had emphasized the necessity for not allowing the circulation in the head to be disturbed by the cold, and insisted on the taking of special precautions in this matter, Bruno insists that wounds must be more carefully looked to in summer than in winter, because "putrefaction is greater in warm than in cold weather"—*putrefactio est major in æstate quam in hyeme*. He is particularly insistent on the necessity of drainage. In wounds of the extremities the limb must always be so placed as to encourage drainage. To secure it the wound may be enlarged; if necessary, even a counter-opening must be made to provide drainage. In order to secure proper union care must be exercised to bring the wound edges accurately together, and not allow hair or oil or dressings to come between them. In large wounds he considers stitching indispensable, and the preferable suture material in his experience is silk or linen. He discusses healing by first and second intention, and declares that with proper care the healing of a great many wounds by first intention can be secured. All his treatment of wounds is dry. Water he considered always did harm, and it is quite easy to understand that his experience taught him this, for the water generally available for surgeons in camps and battlefields and in emergency surgery was likely to do much more harm than good.

Some of the details of his technique of abdominal wounds will be particularly interesting to modern surgeons.

If there was difficulty in bringing about the reposition of the intestines, they were first to be pressed back with a sponge soaked in warm wine. Other manipulations are suggested, and if necessary the wound must be enlarged. If the omentum finds its way out of the wound, all of it that is black or green must be cut off. In cases where the intestines are wounded they are to be sewed with a small needle and a silk thread, and care is to be exercised in bringing about complete closure of the wound. This much will give a good idea of Bruno's thoroughness. Altogether, Gurlt, in his "History of Surgery," gives about fifteen large octavo pages of rather small type to a brief compendium of Bruno's teachings.

One or two other remarks of Bruno are rather interesting in the light of modern development in medicine. For instance, he suggests the possibility of being able to feel a stone in the bladder by means of bimanual palpation. He teaches that mothers may often be able to cure hernias, both umbilical and inguinal, in children by promptly taking up the treatment of them as soon as noticed, bringing the edges of the hernial opening together by bandages, and then preventing the reopening of the hernia, by prohibiting wrestling and loud crying and violent motion. He has seen overgrowth of the mamma in men, and declares that it is due to nothing else but fat, as a rule. He suggests if it should hang down and be in the way on account of its size, it should be extirpated. He seems to have known considerable about the lipomas, and advises that they need only be removed in case they become bothersomely large. The removal is easy, and any bleeding that takes place may be stopped by means of the cautery. He divides rectal fistulæ into penetrating and non-penetrating, and suggests salves for the non-penetrating and the actual cautery for those that penetrate. He warns against the possibility of producing incontinence by the incision of deep fistulæ, for this would leave the patient in a worse state than before.

The most interesting feature of the work of the North Italian surgeons of the later Middle Ages is their discovery and development of the two special advances of our modern surgery in which we are inclined to take most pride. These are, union by first intention, and anæsthesia. It is of course very startling to think that surgeons of seven centuries ago should have made advances in these important phases of surgery—which were afterwards to be forgotten; but human history is not a story of constant progress, but of ups and downs, and the mystery of human history is the decadence that almost inevitably follows any period of supremely great accomplishment by mankind. The later Middle Age enjoyed a particularly great period of efflorescence and achievement in surgery, and this, quite as with literature and other phases of human accomplishment, was followed by distinct descent of interest in surgical theory, and decadence in surgical practice, until the Renaissance came to provide another climax of surgical development. It would be perilous to say, however, that the acme of the curve of Renaissance surgical progress was higher than its predecessor, though once more there is the surprise to find that this high point was followed by another descent, until the curve ascended again in our time.

What we have said already with regard to the requirement of cleanliness in operating upon the skull, insisted upon by the Salernitan School, will suggest that some of the practical value of asepsis had come home to these old-time surgeons. The North Italian surgeons went, however, much farther in their anticipations of asepsis. They insisted that if a surgeon made a wound through an unbroken surface and did not secure union by first intention, it was usually his own fault.

It is to them we owe the expression "union by first intention"—*unio per primam intentionem*—which means nothing to us except through its Latin equivalent. They boasted of getting linear cicatrices which could scarcely be seen, and evidently their practice fostered the best of surgical technique and was founded on excellent principles. The North Italian surgeons replaced the use of ointments by wine, and evidently realized its cleansing—that is, antiseptic—quality. What is often not realized is, that the very old traditional treatment of wounds by the pouring of wine and oil into them represented a mild antiseptic and a soothing protective dressing. The wine inhibited the growth of ordinary germs, the oil protected the wound from dust and dirt. They were not ideal materials for the purpose, but they were much better when discreetly used than many surgical dressings of much more modern times founded on elaborate theories.

Professor Clifford Allbutt, reviewing the practice of these North Italian surgeons of the thirteenth century, says:[9]

"They washed the wound with wine, scrupulously removing every foreign particle; then they brought the edges together, not allowing wine nor anything else to remain within—dry adhesive surfaces were their desire. Nature, they said, produces the means of union in a viscous exudation—or natural balm, as it was afterwards called by Paracelsus, Paré, and Wurtz. In older wounds they did their best to obtain union by cleansing, desiccation, and refreshing of the edges. Upon the outer surface they laid only lint steeped in wine. Powder they regarded as too desiccating, for powder shuts in decomposing matters; wine, after washing, purifying, and drying the raw surfaces, evaporates."

Theodoric wrote in 1266 on that question that so much disturbed the surgeons of the generations before ours, as to whether pus was a natural development in the healing of wounds or not. While laudable pus was for centuries after his time supposedly a scientific doctrine, Theodoric did not think so, and emphatically insisted that such teaching represented a great error. He said: "For it is not necessary, as Roger and Roland have written, as many of their disciples teach, and as all *modern* surgeons profess, that pus should be generated in wounds. No error can be greater than this. Such a practice is indeed to hinder nature, to prolong the disease, and to prevent the conglutination and consolidation of the wound." The italics in the word modern are mine, but the whole expression might well have been used by some early advocate of antisepsis, or even by Lord Lister himself. Just six centuries almost to the year would separate the two declarations, yet they would be just as true at one time as at another. When we learn that Theodoric was proud of the beautiful cicatrices which his father had obtained without the use of any ointment—*pulcherrimas cicatrices sine unguento inducebat*—then, further, that he impugned the use of poultices and of oils in wounds, while powders were too drying, and besides had a tendency to prevent drainage (the literal meaning of the Latin words he employs, *saniem incarcerare*, is to "incarcerate sanious material"), it is easy to understand that the claim that antiseptic surgery was anticipated six centuries ago is no exaggeration and no far-fetched explanation, with modern ideas in mind, of certain clever modes of dressing hit upon accidentally by medieval surgeons.

After Bruno, who brought with him the methods and principles of surgery from the South of Italy, his contemporary of the North, Hugh of Lucca—Ugo da Lucca, or Luccanus, as he is also called—deserves to be mentioned. He was called to Bologna in 1214 as City Physician, and was with the regiment of crusaders from Bologna at Damietta in 1220. He returned to Bologna in 1221 and occupied the post of legal physician. The Civic Statutes of Bologna are, according to Gurlt, the oldest monument of legal medicine in the Middle Ages. Hugh seems to have been deeply intent on chemical experiments, and especially anodyne and anæsthetic drugs. He is said to have been the first to have taught the sublimation of arsenic. Like many another distinguished practitioner of medicine and surgery, he left no writings. All that we know of him and his work, and above all his technique, we owe to the filial devotion of his son Theodoric.

Anæsthesia is perhaps an even greater surprise in the Middle Ages than practical antisepsis. A great many of these surgeons of the time seem to have experimented with substances that might produce anæsthesia. Mandragora was the base of most of these anæsthetics, though a combination with opium seems to have been a favourite. They succeeded apparently, even with such crude means, in producing insensibility to pain without very serious dangers. One of these methods of Da Lucca was by inhalation, and seems to have been in use for a full century. Guy de Chauliac describes the method as it was used in his day, and a paragraph with regard to it will be found in the chapter on Surgeons of the West of Europe. It is quite clear that the extensive operations which are described in their textbooks of surgery at this time could not possibly have been performed, only that the surgeons were able to secure rather a deep and prolonged insensibility to pain. With anæsthesia combined with antisepsis, it is easy to understand how well equipped the surgeons of this time were for the development of their speciality.

The fourth of these great surgeons at the North of Italy was William of Salicet. He was a pupil of Bruno of Longoburgo. Some idea of his practice as a surgeon may be obtained from even the first chapter of his first book. He begins with the treatment of hydrocephalus—or, as he calls it, "water collected in the heads of children newly born." He rejects opening of the head by incision because of the danger of it. He had successfully treated some of these difficult cases, however, by puncturing the scalp and membrane by a cautery, a very small opening being made and fluid being allowed to escape only drop by drop. William did not quote his predecessors much, but depended to a great extent on his own experience. He has many interesting details of technique with regard to the special subject of surgery of the nose, the ear, the mouth; and he did not even hesitate to treat goitre when it grows large, and says that if the sac is allowed to remain it should be thoroughly rubbed over on the inside with "green ointment." He warned "that in this affection many large bloodvessels make their appearance, and they find their way everywhere through the fleshy mass."

A very interesting development of surgery along a line where it would probably be least expected was in plastic surgery. In the first half of the fifteenth century the two Brancas, father and son, performed a series of successful operations for the restoration of the nose particularly, and the son invented a series of similar procedures for the restoration of mutilated lips and ears. The father seems to have built up the nose from other portions of the face, possibly using, as Gurlt suggests, the skin of the forehead, as the Indian surgeons had done, though without any known hint of their work. Fazio, the historian of King Alphonso I. of Naples, who died in 1457, describes the favourite operation of Antonio Branca, the son, who in order not to disfigure any further the face in these cases, made the new nose from the skin of the upper arm; and in anticipation of Tagliacozzi, who attracted much attention by a similar operation in the latter half of the sixteenth century, separated the new nose from the arm sometime during the third week. There is abundance of other evidence as to the Brancas' work from contemporary writers—for instance, Bishop Peter Ranzano the annalist, the poet Calenzio, and Alexander Benedetti, the physician and anatomist—so that there can be no doubt of the fact that this wonderful invention in surgical technique was actually made before the close of the Middle Ages.

It is interesting to realize that, while we hear much about the work of the Brancas, and from ecclesiastical authorities, there is no word of condemnation of the practice of restoring the nose or other facial features until much later in history. Tagliacozzi, who revived the operation of rhinoplasty just about the beginning of the seventeenth century, did not share so kind a fate. The latter Italian surgeon was roundly abused by some of his colleagues, even, it is said, by Fallopius and Paré, and bitterly satirized in Butler's "Hudibras." As late as 1788 (!) the Paris faculty interdicted face-repairing altogether. It is this sort of intolerance, on some superstitious ground or other, that is usually attributed to the Middle Ages. For such events the adjective medieval seems particularly adapted. As a matter of fact, we find comparatively little trace of such intolerance in medieval times; but it is comparatively easy to find the bitterest treatment of fellow-mortals for all sorts of foolish reasons in the seventeenth and eighteenth centuries.

CHAPTER VII

SURGEONS OUTSIDE OF ITALY: SURGEONS OF THE WEST OF EUROPE

"Sciences are made by addition, and it is not possible that the same man should begin and finish them...." "We are like infants at the neck of a giant, for we can see all that the giant sees and something more."—(Guy De Chauliac, Papal Physician to the Popes at Avignon.)

The very interesting and in many ways astonishing development of surgery which occurred in Italy in the twelfth and thirteenth centuries, was followed up by similar developments in the western countries of Europe. France was the first to fall into the line of progress with important advances in surgery, and owes her teaching directly to the Italians; but in Flanders, in England, in Spain, and in Germany, we have records of some significant advances in surgery, and distinguished surgeons wrote books that fortunately for the history of surgery were preserved. The most important of the surgical writings of the time, put in type during the great nascent period of printing at the Renaissance, have come down to us. Many of these have been republished in recent years, and as the texts are now readily available they enable anyone to see for himself just what were the interests of the surgeons of the later medieval period, their technique, and their successful applications of great practical principles to the solution of important surgical problems.

The beginning of French scientific surgery came with the exile from Italy of Lanfranc, as he is known, though his Italian name was Lanfranchi or Lanfranco, and he is sometimes spoken of as Alanfrancus. He had practised as physician and surgeon in Milan until banished from there by Matteo Visconti, about 1290. He made his way then to Lyons, where he attracted so much attention by his success as a surgeon that he was offered the chair of professor of surgery at the University of Paris. "He attracted an almost incredible number of scholars to his lessons in Paris, and by hundreds literally they accompanied him to the bedside of his patient and attended his operations" (Gurlt). Paris was at this time at the very height of its glory as a University. It had had a series of distinguished professors whose writings are still known and honoured, Albert the Great, Thomas Aquinas, Roger Bacon, and Duns Scotus; and during the latter half of the thirteenth century Louis IX. had encouraged the University in every way, and had helped in the foundation of the Sorbonne. There were probably more students in attendance at the University of Paris about the time that Lanfranc was there than there has ever been in attendance at any University before or since. The prestige of Lanfranc's position, then, and his opportunity to impress the world of his time, can be readily appreciated.

The Dean of the medical faculty of Paris, Jean de Passavant, urged Lanfranc to write a textbook of surgery, partly for the familiar academic reason that the students were clamouring for some definite record of his teaching, but also because the Dean felt that the many copies of these lessons which the students would take away with them, and which would be consulted by others, would add greatly to the prestige of the medical school. Medical school officials are not so different after more than six and a half centuries. Lanfranc completed his textbook of surgery, called "Chirurgia Magna," in 1296, and dedicated it to Philippe le Bel, the then reigning King of France. It is from this work that we are able to judge exactly what the value of Lanfranc's surgical teaching was.

In the second chapter of his textbook—the first containing the definition of surgery and a general introduction—Lanfranc devotes some paragraphs to the surgeon himself, and the qualities that a surgeon should possess if he is to be successful in his speciality. It is about the sort of advice that older surgeons are still likely to give young men who are entering on the practice of the speciality, and more or less what is said at many a commencement in the modern time when the maker of the address to the graduates is a surgeon.

"It is necessary that a surgeon should have a temperate and moderate disposition. That he should have well-formed hands, long slender fingers, a strong body, not inclined to tremble, and with all his members trained to the capable fulfilment of the wishes of his mind. He should be well grounded in natural science, and should know not only medicine but every part of philosophy; should know logic well, so as to be able to understand what is written; to talk properly, and to support what he has to say by good reasons." He suggests that it would be well for the surgeon to have spent some time teaching grammar and dialectics and rhetoric, especially if he is to teach others in surgery, for this practice will add greatly to his teaching power. (What a desideratum for the modern time is thus outlined!) Some of his expressions might well be repeated to young surgeons in the modern time. "The surgeon should not love difficult cases, and should not allow himself to be tempted to undertake those that are desperate. He should help the poor as far as he can, but he should not hesitate to ask for good fees from the rich."

Lanfranc was himself a scholar well read in the literature of his profession, but who had well digested his reading. He quotes altogether more than a score of writers on surgery who had preceded him, and evidently was thoroughly familiar with general surgical literature. He is a particular favourite of Gurlt, the German historian of surgery, who has devoted more than twenty-five closely printed large octavo pages to the discussion of this old Paris professor and his work. Lanfranc's discussion of wounds of nerves is of itself sufficient to show the character of his work. Many generations after his time have used the word nerves for tendons, and mistaken the function of these two structures, but Lanfranc distinguished very clearly between them. He declared that since the nerves are instruments of sense and motion, wounds of them should be carefully treated, especially as the sensitiveness of these structures is likely to cause the patient much subsequent pain if they are neglected. Longitudinal wounds of nerves are much less dangerous than those across them. When a nerve is completely divided in cross section Lanfranc was of the opinion, though Theodoric and some others were opposed to it, that the nerve ends should be stitched together. He says that the suture insures the reintegration of the nerve much better. Besides, after this operation the restoration of the usefulness of the member is more assured and is commonly more complete.

After Lanfranc at Paris came Henri de Mondeville, whom Latin writers usually quote as *Henricus*. At least a dozen variants of the second portion of his name are found in literature, from Armondeville to Hermondaville. He was another of the University men of this time who wandered far for opportunities in education. Though born in the North of France and receiving his preliminary education there, he made his medical studies in the latter half of the thirteenth century under Theodoric in Italy. Afterwards he studied medicine in Montpellier and surgery in Paris. Later he gave at least one course of lectures at Montpellier, and then a series of lectures in Paris, attracting to both universities during his professorship a crowd of students from every part of Europe. One of his teachers at Paris had been his compatriot, Jean Pitard, the surgeon of Philippe le Bel, of whom he speaks as "most skilful and expert in the practice of surgery," and it was doubtless to Pitard's friendship that he owed his appointment as one of the four surgeons and three physicians who accompanied the King into Flanders.

There is an historical tradition which has led many to believe that the surgery of the fourteenth century was mainly in the hands of the barber surgeons—ignorant men who plied a rude handicraft in connection with some conventional use of the lancet—and that the physicians quite despised their surgical colleagues. Mondeville is a striking contradiction of this. He was a scholarly man, who quotes not only all the distinguished contributors to medicine and surgery before his time, the Greeks and Latins, the Arabs, and his Italian masters, but who also has quotations from poets and philosophers, Aristotle, Plato, Diogenes, Cato, Horace, Ovid, Seneca, and others.

The Regius Professors of Medicine at both Oxford and Cambridge in our generation are on record with the declaration that medicine and surgery have been allowed to drift too far apart, and that above all the physician should see more of surgical operations for the confirmation of diagnoses, for they are real bioscopys. It is rather interesting to find, then, that Mondeville felt the necessity in his time for close relations between physicians and surgeons, and said:

"It is impossible that a surgeon should be expert who does not know not only the principles, but everything worth while knowing about medicine," and then he added, "just as it is impossible for a man to be a good physician who is entirely ignorant of the art of surgery." He says further: "This our art of surgery, which is the third part of medicine [the other two parts were diet and drugs] is, with all due deference to physicians, considered by us surgeons ourselves and by the non-medical as a more certain, nobler, securer, more perfect, more necessary, and more lucrative art than the other parts of medicine." Surgeons have always been prone to glory in their speciality.

Mondeville is particularly interesting for the history of surgery because he himself ventured to trace some of the recent history of the development of his speciality. Following Galen's example, who had divided the physicians of the world into three sects, the Methodists, the Empirics, and the Rationalists, Mondeville divides modern surgery into three sects: First, that of the Salernitans, with Roger, Roland, and the Four Masters; second, that of William of Salicet, and Lanfranc; and third, that of Ugo da Lucca and his son Theodoric and their modern [*sic*] disciples.

The characteristics of these three sects are in brief. The first limited patients' diet, used no stimulants, dilated all wounds and looked for union only after pus formation. The second allowed a liberal diet to weak patients, though not to the strong, but generally interfered with wounds too much. The third believed in a liberal diet, never dilated wounds, never inserted tents, and its members were extremely careful not to complicate wounds of the head by unwise interference. Almost needless to say, his critical discussion of the three schools is extremely interesting.

Mondeville was himself a broadly educated scholar, who considered that the surgeon should know everything worth while knowing about medicine, for his work was greater than that of the physician. While he had high ideas, however, of the value of theoretic knowledge, he insisted above all on the value of practical training. He said, in his textbook on surgery, as to what the training of the surgeon should be:

"A surgeon who wishes to operate regularly ought first for a long time to frequent places in which skilled surgeons often operate, and he ought to pay careful attention to their operations and commit their technique to memory. Then he ought to associate himself with them in doing operations. A man cannot be a good surgeon unless he knows both the art and science of medicine, and especially anatomy. The characteristics of a good surgeon are that he should be moderately bold, not given to disputations before those who do not know medicine, operate with foresight and wisdom, not beginning dangerous operations until he has provided himself with everything necessary for lessening the danger. He should have well-shaped members, especially hands with long slender fingers, mobile and not tremulous, and with all his members strong and healthy, so that he may perform all the proper operations without disturbance of mind. He must be highly moral, should care for the poor for God's sake, see that he makes himself well paid by the rich, should comfort his patients by pleasant discourse, and should always accede to their requests if these do not interfere with the cure of the disease." "It follows from this," he says, "that the perfect surgeon is more than the perfect physician, and that while he must know medicine he must in addition know his handicraft."

The other great French surgeon of the fourteenth century was Guy de Chauliac, who well deserves the name of father of modern surgery. He was educated in a little town in the South of France, made his medical studies at Montpellier, and then went on a journey of hundreds of miles to Italy in order to make his postgraduate studies. While it is not generally realized, for some seven centuries before the nineteenth Italy was the home of graduate teaching in all departments. Whenever a man in any country in Europe, from the beginning of the twelfth until the end of the eighteenth century, wanted to secure opportunities for the higher education that were not available in his home country, he went down into Italy. At the beginning of the nineteenth century France usurped Italy's place for half a century, and Germany pre-empted the position to a great degree during the latter half of the nineteenth. The journey to Italy in the Middle Ages was more difficult, and involved more expense and time, than would even the voyage from America to Europe in our time; yet many a student from France, Germany, and England made it for the sake of the postgraduate opportunities, and it is matter for professional pride that this was particularly true of our medieval colleagues in medicine and surgery.

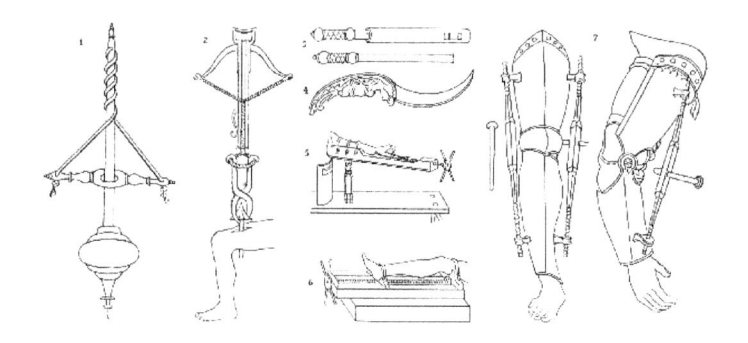

SURGICAL INSTRUMENTS OF GUY DE CHAULIAC, NOS. 1, 2, 3, AND 4 (FOURTEENTH CENTURY);
AND SURGICAL APPARATUS OF HANS VON GERSSDORFF, NOS. 5, 6 AND 7 (FIFTEENTH CENTURY)
After plates in Gurlt's "Geschichte der Chirurgie"

1. Trepan
2. Balista used for extraction of arrows
3. Cauterizing shears with cannula for cauterization of the uvula
4. Bistoury
5. Extension arrangement for reducing upper arm dislocations, called "The Fool"
6. Screwpiece for extending a knee contracture
7. Extension apparatus in the form of armour-arm and armour-leg plates ("harness instruments") for contractures of the elbow and knee joints

To know Guy de Chauliac's works well is to have ready contradictions at hand to practically all of the objections so frequently repeated as to the lack of scholarly work during the Middle Ages. For instance, Guy de Chauliac insisted on the value of experience rather than authority, and of original work rather than mere copying. He criticized in bitter satire John of Gaddesden's book on medicine, called after the fashion of the time by the poetical title "Rosa Anglica," of which he said: "Last of all bloomed the scentless Rose of England, which on its being sent to me I hoped to find bearing the odour of sweet originality. But instead of that I encountered only the fictions of Hispanus, of Gilbert, and of Theodoric." His mode of satirical expression is all the more interesting and significant, because it shows that the men of the time were critically minded enough as regards many of the passages in the writings of their predecessors with which fault has been found in the modern time, though we have usually been inclined to think that medieval readers accepted them quite uncritically. Chauliac's bitterest reproach for many of his predecessors was that "they follow one another like cranes, whether for love or fear I cannot say."

Chauliac's description of the methods of anæsthesia practised by the surgeons of his time, especially in cases of amputation, is particularly interesting to us because the anæsthetic was administered by inhalation. Chauliac says:

"Some surgeons prescribe medicaments, such as opium, the juice of the morel, hyoscyamus, mandrake, ivy, hemlock, lettuce, which send the patient to sleep, so that the incision may not be felt. A new sponge is soaked by them in the juice of these and left to dry in the sun; when they have need of it they put this sponge into warm water, and then hold it under the nostrils of the patient until he goes to sleep. Then they perform the operation."[10]

Chauliac was particularly interested in the radical cure of hernia, and he discusses six different operations for this purpose. Gurlt points out that Chauliac's criticism of these operations is quite modern in its viewpoint. He declared that practically the object of radical operations for hernia is to produce a strong, firm tissue support over the ring through which the cord passes, so that the intestines cannot descend through it. It is rather interesting to find that the surgeons of this time tried to obliterate the canal by means of the cautery, or inflammation-producing agents—arsenic and the like—a practice that recalls some methods still used more or less irregularly. They also used gold wire as a support; it was to be left in the tissues, and was supposed to protect and strengthen the closure of the ring. At this time all these operations for the radical cure of hernia involved the sacrifice of the testicle, because the old surgeons wanted to obliterate the ring completely, and thought this the easiest way. Chauliac criticizes the operation in this respect, but says that he has "seen many cases in which men possessed of but one testicle have procreated, and this is a problem where the lesser of two evils is to be chosen."

While he discussed hernia operations so freely, the great French surgeon did not believe that everyone who suffered from a hernia ought to be submitted to an operation. He quite agreed with Mondeville who, in the preceding generation, declared that many operations for hernia were done not for the benefit of the patient but for the benefit of the surgeon—a mode of expression that is likely to strike a sympathetic chord in some physicians' minds even at the present time. Chauliac's rule was that no operation should be attempted unless the patient's life was put in danger by the hernia, but that a truss should be worn to retain it. He emphasized that trusses should not be made according to rule, but must be adapted to each individual, and he invented several forms of trusses himself. He developed the method of taxis by which hernias might be reduced, suggested an exaggerated Trendelenburg position for operations for hernia and for the manipulations necessary for the reduction of hernia.

The technique of some of these old surgeons is a never-ending source for surprise. The exaggerated Trendelenburg position in the operation for the radical cure of hernia—the patient being fastened on an inclined board, head down, so that the intestines would fall away from the site of operation—was used by Guy de Chauliac, who probably obtained a hint of it from Italy. He also employed extension in the treatment of fracture of the thigh, inventing an apparatus by which this might be continued for a long time until the muscles were relaxed from overtiredness. He made use for this purpose of a weight suspended on a cord which ran over rollers. He also adapted stiffened bandages of various kinds, especially employing white of egg for this, and sometimes moulding bandages to the limbs in cases of fracture. Yperman, the Flemish surgeon of this time, knew and used the œsophagus tube for artificial feeding, and a number of various kinds of instruments were invented for the urethra, including bougies of wax, tin, and silver. In diseases of the bladder and in gonorrhœa John Ardern employed astringent injections.

Probably what ought to be considered the most important work of the French surgeons of the Middle Ages has been quite misunderstood until recent years. In his paper on "The Origin of Syphilis," at the Seventeenth International Congress of Medicine (London, 1913), Professor Karl Südhoff of Leipzig (see Transactions) reviewed the use of mercury in the form of mercurial ointment during the later Middle Ages, and the reputation that it had acquired for the cure of ulcers, skin eruptions of various kinds, and other distinctly objective lesions. It is perfectly clear now that the success of this form of therapy was due to the fact that syphilis was being treated. The French surgeons of the South of France developed the empiric discovery of the value of this remedy, the first hint of which had probably come to them from the Italians. It is one of the few specifics in the history of medicine. Needless to say, it is still with us, and still the accepted medication in spite, as Professor Südhoff notes, of the often-attempted replacement of it down the centuries by some form or other of arsenic treatment, though this has always been afterwards abandoned, and it would seem as though our generation might furnish another instance of the triumph of the medieval mercurial treatment over arsenic.

The real reason then, it would seem, why syphilis came to be called the *morbus Gallicus*, or French Disease, was because when knowledge of its differential diagnosis was generalized, physicians at the same time learned of the remedy which could be so successfully employed for its treatment, the value of which had been determined as the result of the careful observations of the surgeons of South France. It is probable, as I have said, that the original idea for this form of treatment came from the Italian surgical traditions brought over from Italy by Lanfranc and his contemporaries at the end of the thirteenth century. There can be no doubt at all, however, of the power of clinical observation of the medieval surgeons who gave us this wonderful advance in therapeutics.

The most distinguished pupil of Guy de Chauliac was Pietro d'Argelata, who died about 1423 as a professor at Bologna, but whose textbook, "The Cirurgia," was among the first of medical books to be printed at Venice in 1480. His teaching was still a living force at that time, and it is evident that he had attracted wide attention in his own generation. He taught the dry treatment of wounds, suggesting various powders to be employed on them, and gave his experience with sutures and drainage tubes in wounds.

Ligatures are often supposed to have been invented much later. They have been attributed to Ambroise Paré and other surgeons of the Renaissance period, but were probably used at many times during the Middle Ages, and had been invented and frequently employed by the Greeks. They invariably went out of use after a time, however, and had to be reinvented. As I said in "Old-Time Makers of Medicine":

"It is hard to understand how so useful an auxiliary to the surgeon as the ligature—it seems indispensable to us—could possibly be allowed to go out of use and even be forgotten. It will not be difficult, however, for anyone who recalls the conditions that obtained in old-time surgery to understand the succession of events. The ligature is a most satisfying immediate resource in stopping bleeding from an artery, but a septic ligature inevitably causes suppuration, and almost inevitably leads to secondary hæmorrhage. In the old days of septic surgery, secondary hæmorrhage was the surgeon's greatest and most dreaded bane. Some time from the fifth to the ninth day a septic ligature came away under conditions such that inflammatory disturbance had prevented sealing of the vessel. If the vessel was large, the hæmorrhage was fast and furious, and the patient died in a few minutes. After a surgeon had had a few deaths of this kind he dreaded the ligature.

"Eventually he abandoned its use, and took kindly even to such methods as the actual cautery, red-hot knives for amputations and the like, that would sear the surfaces of tissues, and the bloodvessels, and not give rise to secondary hæmorrhage. A little later, however, someone not familiar with the secondary risks would reinvent the ligature. If he were cleanly in his methods, and, above all, if he were doing his work in a new hospital, the ligature worked very well for a while. If not, it soon fell into innocuous desuetude again. In any case, it was only a question of time until it would be abandoned."

There was at least one, and probably a number of English surgeons who were doing excellent work in the latter part of the Middle Ages, but John of Ardern wrote a book which has come down to us, and from him we may judge the character of his contemporaries. He was educated at Montpellier, and practised surgery for a time in France. About the middle of the fourteenth century, according to Pagel, he went back to his native land and settled for some twenty years at Newark in Nottinghamshire; and for nearly thirty years longer, until near the end of the century, practised in London. Ardern's speciality was diseases of the rectum, but he made special studies in the treatment of fistulas everywhere in the body. He was an expert operator, and seems to have had excellent success in this field. He made careful statistics of his cases, and was quite as proud as any modern surgeon of the large numbers that he had operated on, which he gives very exactly. He was the inventor of some new instruments and of a clyster apparatus. We know something also about his fees, and there is no doubt that he obtained quite as good fees in proportion to the value of money as even any specialist of the modern time.

Ardern gives many evidences of his power of clinical observation, and incidentally makes it very clear that the eyes of the men of his time were not so held from seeing the things that lay before them as is often assumed. Mr. D'Arcy Power, in the paper on "The Lesser Writings of John Ardern" which he read before the section on the History of Medicine at the Seventeenth International Congress (see Transactions), has quoted a series of paragraphs from Ardern which make it very clear how accurate an observer this fourteenth-century Englishman was. Here, for instance, is his description of epidemic sore throat in his time, probably diphtheria, for the death within five days through strangling would seem to point to this:

"And note diligently that in the sqwynancy [quinsy] and in all the swellynges of the throte and the nekke and in all the lettynges and swolowynge as whanne the pacient thereof is oftetymys dysposyd to the deeth withinne schort time and I have seye manye deyed thereof within v dayes thorough stranglynge. To the weche it is to know that ther is nothynge more profytablere therefore thane to use glysteryes of malowys, mercurye [cheno-podium?] branne and oyle or buttre, hony and Sal gemme or comone salt. This operacione draweth the wykkyd humours to the inner partyes that causeth the syknesse and so it helpeth the sqwynnancye."

Ardern's description of rabies, its fatality, and of how a mad dog acts, exemplifies still further his accuracy of clinical observation. Only one who had seen many cases and understood them, and had had many mad dogs under observation, could have given the details he does. A single paragraph confirms the idea that the medieval surgeons had very clearly recognized the disease, and knew as much about it as was known until our own generation added something of more definite knowledge of the affection than could be gained by mere clinical observation. Ardern says:

"The bytynge of a wood [mad] dogge is more venemous and perilous thane it is of a serpente, ffor the venyme of a wood dogge ys hydd often tymes by the hole yere togydere and other whyle by the ii [two] yere and after some auctours it wole endure vii yere or it sle [slay] a man. And note wheyther it be longe tyme hydd or schorte or that it slee ther comene tofore to the pacient thes tokenys medlynge and chaungynge of wytte and resone and abhominacione and lothsomnesse of cold water that is clene and pure. And whane suche sygnys fallen to him that is byten of a wood hound schall unnethe or ellys [seldom or never] escape it.

"The tokenys of a wood dogge ben these; the furste is he knoweth not his lord ne his mayster and he falleth into a voyd goyinge allone with boowynge of his heed and hangynge of the erys [ears] as other wyse than ne he hadde hemin his helthe and the yene [eyes] of him ben rede and the fome cometh out at the mowth and he wole berke at his oune schadowe and he hath ane hos [hoarse] berkynge, and other houndes fleene from hyme and berken towardys hyme. And yf a schyvere [slice] of breed be folden or wette in the bytynge of the sore and yoven a dogge to ete, yf that he ete it, it is a token that the dogge is not wood, for and the dogge be wood tha other dogge that the breed is yoven to wole not ete it, but that he be over moche hungry, and yf he denye to ete the seyde breed, out-take [unless on] the condicione aforeseyd, thane is the dogge wood."

Ardern's description of a case of traumatic tetanus is very interesting, because it contains so many elements that are familiar in the history of this affection. The fact that it occurred in a gardener from a hook, so likely to be infected with tetanus bacilli from hay or grass, and that the wound was made where the thumb joins the hand and where, as we know now, the construction of the tissues is so favourable to that burying of the tetanus bacilli away from the free oxygen of the air, giving it a chance to grow anaerobically, all show the disease exactly as in our own time. The other details of the case probably indicate a wound of an important bloodvessel, secondary hæmorrhage after suppuration had been established, and then the development of fatal subacute tetanus.

"A gardinere whyle that he wrowghte in the vynes kytte his owne hande with ane hooke uppone a ffryday after the ffeste of Seynt Thomas of Caunterbury in somere so that the thoombe was altogydere departyd from the hande saff only in the juncture that was joyned to the hande, and he myghte boowe bakward the thoombe to his arme and ther stremyd out therof moche blood.

"And so touchynge to the cure. The thoombe was furst reduced in to his furste ordre and sowyd and the blood was restreyned with the reed pouder of launfrankes [Lanfranc's red powder] and with the heerys [hairs] of ane hare and it was not remevyd une-to the iiide day when it was remevyd tther apperyd no blood. Thanne was ther putte therto tho medicines that engendren blood, every day ones repeyrynge the wounde, and tho it began to purge itselffe and to gadere mater. And in the iiiithe nyght after the blood brak out abowte mydnyght in the wheyghte of ii poundes. And whane the blod was restreyned the wounde was repeyred frome day to day as it was furste.

"Also in the xithe nyght abowte the forseyd oure the blood brake owt ayene [again] in more quantyte thane it dyde afore tyme, nevertheless the blood was staunched, and by the morne the pacient was so taken with the crampe in the chekes [cheeks] and in the arme that he myght resseyve no mete in-to his mowth ne neyther opene the mowyth (lockjaw) and so vexynge the pacient in the xv day the blood brake out ayene owt of mesure and alwey the crampe endured forth and in the xx day he dyde."

Another important surgeon of the West of Europe whose book has come down to us was John Yperman, who owes his name to the fact that he was a native of the town of Ypres (in Flemish Ypern) in Flanders. Yperman was sent by his fellow-townsmen to Paris in order to study surgery, apparently at the expense of the municipality, because they wanted to have a good surgeon in their town, and Paris seemed the best school at that time. Ypres, so familiar now as the scene of bloody battles, had become even before the war one of the less important cities even of Belgium, with less than 20,000 people. It was in the thirteenth century one of the greatest commercial cities of Europe, and probably had several hundred thousand inhabitants. The great hall of the Cloth Guild, one of the architectural triumphs of the time, and such an attraction for visitors to the town ever since (destroyed in the war) was built at this time, and is another tribute to the community feeling of the citizens, who determined upon the very sensible procedure of assuring the best possible surgery for themselves and fellow-citizens by having one of their townsmen specially educated for that purpose. Yperman's book on surgery was well known in his own time, but remained unprinted until about half a century ago (1854), when Carolus of Ghent issued an edition. Subsequent editions were issued by Broeckx, the Belgian historian (Antwerp, 1863), and by van Leersum (1913), who gathered some details of the great Flemish surgeon's life. After his return from Paris, Yperman obtained great renown, which maintains in the custom extant in that part of the country even yet of calling an expert surgeon "an Yperman." He is the author of two works in Flemish. One of these is a smaller compendium of internal medicine, which is very interesting, however, because it shows the many subjects that were occupying physicians' minds at that time. He treats of dropsy, rheumatism, under which occur the terms coryza and catarrh (the flowing diseases), icterus, phthisis (he calls the tuberculous, tysiken), apoplexy, epilepsy, frenzy, lethargy, fallen palate, cough, shortness of breath, lung abscess, hæmorrhage, blood-spitting, liver abscess, hardening of the spleen, affections of the kidney, bloody urine, diabetes, incontinence of urine, dysuria, strangury, gonorrhœa, and involuntary seminal emissions—all these terms are quoted directly from Pagel's account of his work.

There is not much to be said of the surgery of Germany during the Middle Ages, though toward the end of this period a series of important documents for the history of surgery were written which serve to show how much was being accomplished, though the subsequent religious and political disturbances in Germany doubtless led to the destruction of many other documents that would have supplied valuable information. Heinrich von Pfolspeundt's book, which is a work on bandaging—"Bundth-Ertzney"—was published in 1460, and the experience for it was therefore all obtained in the Middle Ages. While its main purpose is bandaging, it contains many hints of the surgical knowledge of the time. There are chapters devoted to injuries and wounds, though it is distinctly stated that the book is for "wound physicians" (*Wund Aertzte*) and not for cutting physicians (*Schneide Aertzte*)—that is, for those who do operations apart from wounds. There are two operations described, however, that have particular interest. One of them involves the plastic surgery of the nose, and the other the repair of a hare-lip.

Pfolspeundt suggested that stitches should be placed on the mucous surface as well as on the skin surface, after the edges of the cleft in hare-lip had been freshened in order to be brought closely together for healing with as little deformity as possible. Perhaps his most interesting surgical hint for us is a description of a silver tube with flanges to be inserted in the intestines whenever there were large wounds, or when the intestines had been divided. The ends of the gut were brought together carefully over the tube and stitched together, the tube being allowed to remain *in situ*. Pfolspeundt says that he had often seen these tubes used and the patient live for many years afterwards. While this resembles some of the mechanical aids to surgery of the intestines that have been suggested in our time, this was not the first mechanical device of this kind that had been thought of. One of the later medieval surgeons in Italy, one of the

Brancas, had employed the trachea of an animal as the tube over which the wounded intestines were brought together. This had the advantage of not having to be passed, for after a time it became disintegrated in the secretions, but it remained intact until after thorough agglutination of the intestines had occurred.

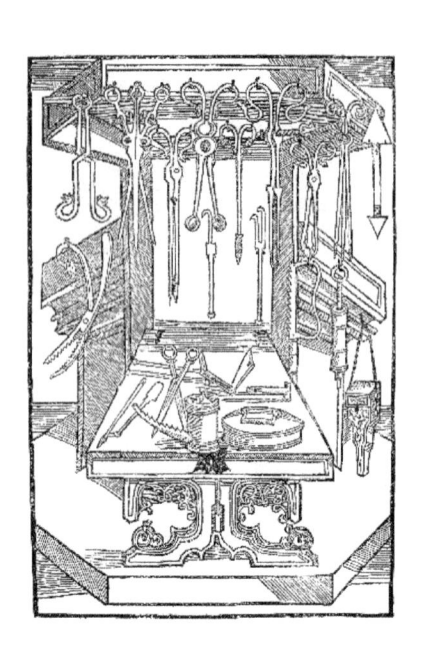

BRUNSCHWIG'S SURGICAL ARMAMENTARIUM
From Gurlt's "Geschichte der Chirurgie"

Hans von Gerssdorff and Hieronymus Brunschwig, who flourished in the latter half of the fifteenth century in Germany, have both left early printed treatises on Surgery which give excellent woodcuts showing pictures of instruments, operations, and costumes, at the end of the medieval period.

CHAPTER VIII

ORAL SURGERY AND THE MINOR SURGICAL SPECIALITIES

The surgical specialities, as they are called—that is, the surgery of the mouth, throat, and nose, and of the eye and ear, as well of course as of certain other portions of the body—have developed to a striking extent in our time. As a consequence of this recent development, there is an impression prevalent that this is the first time that serious attention has been paid by surgeons to these phases of their work. The feeling is probably that the minor operations usually required in the surgical specialities were either thought so trivial, or involved such delicate technique, that they never received due attention, rather than that they were deliberately neglected.

Because of this very general persuasion, even among physicians, it is all the more interesting to trace the phases of attention during the Middle Ages to these special subjects in surgery, which was far from lacking at any time, and which led at various periods to some rather important developments. While specialism is considered new by most people, it must not be forgotten that at every time in the world's history, when men have had much chance to think about themselves rather than the actual necessities of the situation in which they were placed, and the things they were compelled to do for actual self-preservation, specialism has enjoyed a period of more or less intense evolution. It is rather easy to trace this in the Ebers Papyrus near the beginning of the second millennium B.C.; and Herodotus called attention to the fact that the old Egyptians had divided the practice of medicine into many specialities. His passage on the subject is well known.[11]

If the surgical specialities had been neglected in the Middle Ages, then that fact would have constituted the surest evidence of that backwardness of medical and surgical progress which is usually supposed to have existed at that time. But the real story is exactly to the contrary, and has many surprises in it because of the anticipations of very recent advances which it represents.[12]

It would be surprising, then, if we were to find no attention paid to dentistry during the Middle Ages. As a matter of fact, a number of the old surgeons include in their textbooks of surgery the discussion of oral surgery. Aëtius evidently knew much about the hygiene of the teeth, and discusses extraction and the cure of fistulæ of the gums as well as the surgical treatment of many other lesions of the mouth. Paul of Ægina in the century after Aëtius has even more details; and while they both quote mainly from older authors, there seems no doubt that they themselves must have had considerable practical experience in the treatment of the teeth and had made not a few observations. The Arabians took up the subject, and discussed dental diseases and their treatment rationally and in considerable detail. Abulcassis particularly has much that is of significance and interest. We have pictures of two score of dental instruments that were used by him. The Arabs not only treated and filled carious teeth, and even replaced those that were lost, but they also corrected deformities of the mouth and the dental arches. Orthodontia is usually thought of as of much later origin, yet no one who knows Abulcassis's work can speak of efforts at straightening the teeth as *invented* after his time.

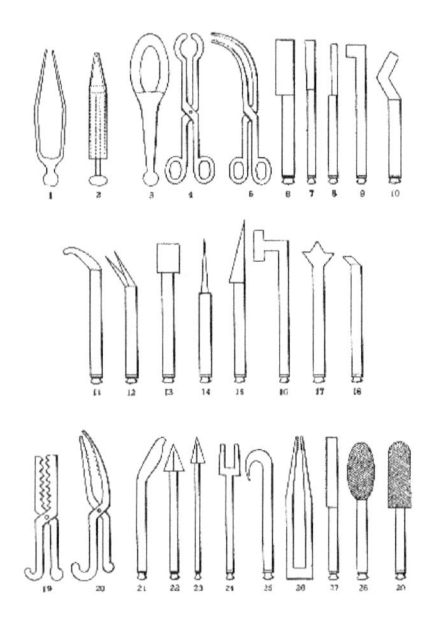

SURGICAL INSTRUMENTS OF THE ARABS, ACCORDING TO ABULCASIM
After plates in Gurlt's "Geschichte der Chirurgie"

1. A pincher for extracting foreign bodies from the ear

2. An ear syringe for injections

3. A tongue depressor

4. Concave scissors for the removal of tonsils

5. Curved pinchers for foreign bodies in the throat

6 to 29. Instruments for the treatment of the teeth

19 and 20. Forceps

21 to 25. Levers and hooks for the removal of roots

26. Strong pinchers for the same

27. A tooth saw 28 and 29. Files for the teeth

The great surgeons of the later Middle Ages in their textbooks of surgery usually include remarks on oral surgery, and suggest treatment for the various diseases of the teeth. Guy de Chauliac in "La Grande Chirurgie" lays down certain rules for the preservation of the teeth, and shows that the ordinary causes of dental decay were well recognized in his time. Emphasis was laid by him on not taking foods too hot or too cold, and above all on the advisability of not having either hot or cold food followed by something very different from it in temperature. The breaking of hard things with the teeth was warned against as responsible for such fissures in the enamel as gave opportunity for the development of decay. The eating of sweets, and especially the sticky sweets, preserves, and the like, were recognized as an important source of caries. The teeth were supposed to be cleaned frequently, and not to be cleaned too roughly, for this would do more harm than good.

Chauliac is particularly emphatic in his insistence on not permitting alimentary materials to remain in the cavities, and suggests that if cavities between the teeth tend to retain food material they should even be filled in such a way as to prevent these accumulations. His directions for cleansing the teeth were rather detailed. His favourite treatment for wounds was wine, and he knew that he succeeded by means of it in securing union by first intention. It is not surprising, then, to find that he recommends rinsing of the mouth with wine as a precaution against dental decay. A vinous decoction of wild mint and of pepper he considered particularly beneficial, though he thought that dentifrices, either powder or liquid, should also be used. He seems to recommend the powder dentifrices as more efficacious. His favourite prescription for a tooth-powder, while more elaborate, resembles to such an extent at least, some, if not indeed most, of those that are used at the present time, that it seems worth while giving his directions for it. He took equal parts of cuttle-bones, small white seashells, pumice-stone, burnt stag's horn, nitre, alum, rock salt, burnt roots of iris, aristolochia, and reeds. All of these substances should be carefully reduced to powder and then mixed.

His favourite liquid dentifrice contained the following ingredients: Half a pound each of sal ammoniac and rock salt, and a quarter of a pound of saccharin alum. All these were to be reduced to powder and placed in a glass alembic and dissolved. The teeth should be rubbed with it, using a little scarlet cloth for the purpose. Just why this particular colour of cleansing cloth was recommended is not quite clear.

He recognized, however, that cleansing of the teeth properly often became impossible by any scrubbing method, no matter what the dentifrice used, because of the presence of what he called hardened limosity or limyness (*limosité endurcie*). When that condition is present he suggests the use of rasps and spatumina and other instrumental means very similar to those we make use of for removing tartar.

Guy de Chauliac was also interested in mechanical dentistry and the artificial replacement of lost teeth; and, indeed, dental prosthesis represents, as treated by him, a distinct anticipation of dental procedures usually thought quite modern.

When teeth become loose he advises that they be fastened to the healthy ones with a gold chain. Guerini, in his "History of Dentistry" (Philadelphia, 1907), suggests that he evidently means a gold wire. If the teeth fall out Chauliac recommends that they be replaced by the teeth of another person, or with artificial teeth made from ox-bone, which may be fixed in place by a fine metal ligature. He says that such teeth may be serviceable for a long while. This is a rather curt way of treating so large a subject as dental prosthesis, but it contains a lot of suggestive material. He was quoting mainly the Arabian authors, and especially Abulcassis and Ali Abbas and Rhazes—and these of course, as we have said, mentioned many methods of artificially replacing teeth, as also of transplantation and of treatment of the deformities of the dental arches.

Guerini called particular attention to the fact that Chauliac recognized the dentists as specialists. He observes that operations on the teeth are in a class by themselves, and belong to the *dentatores* to whom they had been entrusted. He remarks, however, that the operations on the mouth should be performed under the direction of a surgeon. It is in order to give surgeons the general principles by means of which they may be able to judge of the advisability or necessity for dental operations, that his brief presentation of the subject is made. If their advice is to be of value, physicians should know the various methods of treatment suitable for dental diseases, including "mouth washes, gargles, masticatories and ointments, rubbings, fumigations, cauterizations, fillings, filings," as well as the various dental operations. He says that the *dentator* must be provided with appropriate instruments, among which he named scrapers, rasps, straight and curved, spatumina, elevators, simple and with two branches, toothed tenacula, and many different forms of probes and cannulas. He should have also small scalpels, tooth trephines, and files.

After Guy de Chauliac, the most important contributor to dentistry is Giovanni of Arcoli—or simply Arcolano, but sometimes better known by his Latin name Johannes Arculanus—who was Professor of Medicine and Surgery at Bologna just before and after the middle of the fifteenth century. He is sometimes treated in history as belonging rather to the Renaissance, but he owed his training to the

Middle Ages and was teaching before they closed, so he has a place in Medieval Medicine. Guerini, in his "History of Dentistry," says that Arculanus treats the subject of dentistry rather fully and with great accuracy. The Italian historian makes a summary of Arculanus's rules for dental hygiene which shows how thoroughly he appreciated the care of the teeth. The medieval surgeon arranged his rules in ten distinct canons, creating in this way a kind of decalogue of dental hygiene.

These rules are: (1) It is necessary to guard against the corruption of food and drink within the stomach; therefore, easily corruptible food—milk, salt fish, etc.—must not be partaken of, and after meals all excessive movement, running exercises, bathing, coitus, and other causes that impair the digestion, must also be avoided. (2) Everything must be avoided that may provoke vomiting. (3) Sweet and viscous food—such as dried figs, preserves made with honey, etc.—must not be partaken of. (4) Hard things must not be broken with the teeth. (5) All food, drink, and other substances that set the teeth on edge must be avoided, and especially the rapid succession of hot and cold, and *vice versa*. (7) Leeks must not be eaten, as such a food, by its own nature, is injurious to the teeth. (8) The teeth must be cleaned at once after every meal from the particles of food left in them; and for this purpose thin pieces of wood should be used, somewhat broad at the ends, but not sharp-pointed or edged; and preference should be given to small cypress-twigs, or the wood of aloes, or pine, rosemary, or juniper, and similar sorts of wood, which are rather bitter and styptic; care must, however, be taken not to search too long in the dental interstices, and not to injure the gums or shake the teeth. (9) After this it is necessary to rinse the mouth, using by preference a vinous decoction of sage, or one of cinnamon, mastich, gallia, moschata, cubeb, juniper seeds, root of cyperus, and rosemary leaves. (10) The teeth must be rubbed with suitable dentifrices before going to bed, or else in the morning before breakfast. Although Avicenna recommended various oils for this purpose, Giovanni of Arcoli appears very hostile to oleaginous frictions, because he considers them very injurious to the stomach. He observes, besides, that whilst moderate frictions of brief duration are helpful to the teeth, strengthen the gums, prevent the formation of tartar, and sweeten the breath, too rough or too prolonged rubbing is, on the contrary, harmful to the teeth, and makes them liable to many diseases.

Shortly after Arculanus, when the Middle Ages are over—if they end with the middle of the fifteenth century, though perhaps not if the later date of the discovery of America is to be taken as the medieval terminal—John de Vigo has in a few lines a very complete description of the method of filling teeth with gold-leaf which deserves to be quoted. Only that it was a common practice he would surely have described it more in detail, though he could have added nothing to the significance of what he has to say: "By means of a drill or file the putrefied or corroded part of the teeth should be completely removed. The cavity left should then be filled with gold-leaf."

Much more is known about the medieval anticipation of other specialities—those of the throat and nose, and eye and ear—and the surprise is with regard to dentistry, which is usually quite unknown. The fact, however, that dentistry developed so much more than is usually thought prepares the mind for the anticipations in other departments. Following that of dentistry should come naturally the mouth and throat, and it happens that the men whose writings in dentistry are known also touched on these subjects.

The medical writers of the early Middle Ages, particularly Aëtius, Alexander of Tralles, and Paul of Ægina, have not a little to say with regard to affections of the throat and nose, and the eye and ear. Alexander's chapter on the Treatment of Affections of the Ear, Gurlt considers ample evidence of large practical experience and power of observation. Alexander describes the ordinary mode of getting water out of the external auditory canal by standing on the leg corresponding to the side in which the water is, and kicking out with the opposite leg. Foreign bodies should be removed by an ear spoon, or a small instrument wrapped in wool and dipped in sticky material. He suggests sneezing with the head leaning toward the side on which the foreign body is present. Insects or worms that find their way into the ear may be killed by injections of dilute acid and oil or other substances.

Paul of Ægina has a very practical technique for the removal of fish-bones or other objects caught in the throat. He also gives the detailed technique of opening the larynx or trachea, with the indications for this operation. He also describes how wounds of the neck should be sewed after attempts at suicide. In a word, the more one knows of these old-time medieval writers of the sixth and seventh centuries the clearer it becomes that they had learned their lessons well from the ancients, and passed on an excellent tradition to their colleagues of succeeding generations. If these lessons were not properly taken, it was because the disturbance of civilization caused by the coming down of the Teutonic invaders into Italy took away interest in the things of the mind and of the body, until the coming of another upward turn in progress.

Arculanus has some very interesting paragraphs with regard to the treatment of conditions in the nose. For instance, in the treatment of polyps, he says that they should be incised and cauterized. Soft polyps should be drawn out with a toothed tenaculum as far as can be without risk of breaking them off. The incision should be made at the root, so that nothing or just as little as possible of the pathological structure be allowed to remain. It should be cut off with fine scissors; or with a narrow file just small enough to permit ingress into the nostrils; or with a scalpel without cutting edges on the sides, but only at its extremity, and this cutting edge should be broad and well sharpened. If there is danger of hæmorrhage, or if there is fear of it, the instruments with which the section is made should be fired (*igniantur*)—that is, heated at least to a dull redness. Afterwards the stump, if any remains, should be touched with a hot iron or else with cauterizing agents, so that as far as possible it should be obliterated.

After the operation, a pledget of cotton dipped in the green ointment described by Rhazes should be placed in the nose. This pledget should have a string fastened to it, hanging from the nose, in order that it may be easily removed. At times it may be necessary to touch the root of the polyp with a stylet, on which cotton has been placed that has been dipped in *aqua fortis* (nitric acid). It is important that this cauterizing fluid should be rather strong, so that after a certain number of touches a rather firm eschar is produced. In all these manipulations in the nose Arculanus recommends that the nose should be held well open by means of a nasal speculum. Pictures of all these instruments occur in his extant works, and indeed this constitutes one of their most interesting and valuable features. They are to be seen in Gurlt's "History of Surgery."

In some of the cases he had seen, the polyp was so difficult to get at, or was situated so far back in the nose, that it could not be reached by means of a tenaculum or scissors, or even the special knife devised for that purpose. For these patients Arculanus describes an operation that is to be found in the older writers on surgery—Paul of Ægina (Æginetas), Avicenna, and some of the other Arabian surgeons. For this, three horse-tail hairs are twisted together and knotted in three or four places, and one end is passed through the nostrils and out through the mouth. The ends of this are then pulled on backward and forward after the fashion of a saw. Arculanus remarks, evidently with the air of a man who has tried it and not been satisfied, that this operation is quite uncertain, and seems to depend a great deal on chance, and much reliance must not be placed on it. Arculanus suggests a substitute method by which latent polyps—or occult polyps, as he calls them—may be removed.

Among the affections of the upper air passages mentioned by Arculanus are various forms of sore throat, which he calls Synanche or Cynanche, or angina. A milder form of the affection was called Parasynanche. The medieval teaching with regard to an angina that was causing severe difficulty of breathing was to perform tracheotomy. Arculanus goes into some detail with regard to affections of the uvula, which was made much more responsible for throat affections than at the present time. The popular tradition in our time of the uvula and its fall is evidently a remnant of the medieval teaching with regard to it. Arculanus's description of the removal of the uvula, or at least of the tip of it, gives a very good idea of how thorough the teaching of surgical technique was in his time. His directions are: "Seat the patient upon a stool in a bright light, while an assistant holds the head; after the tongue has been firmly depressed by means of a speculum, let the assistant hold this speculum in place. With the left hand then insert an instrument, a stilus, by which the uvula is pulled forward; and then remove the end of it by means of a heated knife or some other process of cauterization. The mouth should afterwards be washed out with fresh milk."

The application of a cauterizing solution by means of a cotton swab wrapped round the end of a sound may be of service in patients who refuse the actual cautery. To be successful, he insists that the application must be firmly made and must be frequently repeated.

With regard to ophthalmology the older history has always been thoroughly appreciated. Even as early as the time of Hammurabi (2200 B.C.) some rather extensive and interesting surgery of the eye was practised, for the fees for these operations are mentioned in the code. All of the early medieval writers on medicine and surgery—Aëtius, Alexander of Tralles, and Paul of Ægina—have paragraphs at least, and sometimes more, with regard to eye operations and the care of the eyes.

Operations above all for cataract have been practised from very early times, and are mentioned also by many medieval writers on medicine and surgery. It is not surprising, then, to find that the medieval surgeons particularly discussed a number of eye diseases and the operations for them. Pope John XXI., who before he became Pope was known as *Petrus Hispanus* (the Spaniard), and who had been a professor of surgery and a papal physician, wrote a book on eye diseases in the latter half of the thirteenth century, which has come down to us. He had much to say of cataract, dividing it into traumatic and spontaneous, and suggesting operation by needling, a gold needle being used for that purpose. Pope John describes a form of hardness of the eye which would seem to be what we now call glaucoma, and has a number of external applications for eye diseases. Most of his collyria had some bile in them, the bile of various kinds of animals and birds being supposed to be progressively more efficient for the cure of external affections of the eye. This very general use of bile, or of an extract of the livers of animals or fishes, seems to be a heritage from biblical times, when old Toby was cured of his blindness by the gall of the fish.[13] The Pope ophthalmologist (see *Opthalmology*, Milwaukee, January, 1909) recommended the urine of infants as an eye-wash, experience having evidently shown that this fluid, which is usually bland and unirritating, a solution of salts of a specific gravity such that it would not set up osmotic processes in the eye, was empirically of value. In the Middle Ages the idea of using it would be much less deterrent, because it was quite a common practice for physicians to taste urine in order to test it for pathological conditions.

Spectacles were rather commonly used in the Middle Ages, probably having been invented in the second half of the thirteenth century by Salvino de Armato of Florence. Bernard de Gordon mentions them under the name *oculus berellinus* early in the fourteenth century. They were originally made from a kind of smoky crystal, *berillus*, whence the German name *Brillen* and the French *besicles* (Garrison). Guy de Chauliac suggests that when collyria failed to improve the sight spectacles should be employed. Almost needless to say, this use of spectacles meant very much for the comfort and convenience of old people. Up to that time most of those who reached the age of three-score would be utterly unable to read, and would have to depend either on others or on their memory for teaching and many other purposes. External eye troubles, as those due to trichiasis and to various disturbances of the lachrymal apparatus, were treated by direct mechanical means. Some very ingenious suggestions and manipulations were made with regard to them.

CHAPTER IX

MEDICAL EDUCATION FOR WOMEN

Among the rather startling surprises that have developed, as the growth of our knowledge of medieval history, through consultation of the documents in recent years, is constantly contradicting traditions founded on lack of information, perhaps the greatest has been to learn that women were given opportunities for the higher education at practically all of the Italian universities, and that they became not only students, but professors, at many of these institutions. No century from the twelfth down to the nineteenth was without some distinguished women professors at Italian universities, and in the later Middle Ages there was a particularly active period of feminine education.

The most interesting feature of this development for us is that the application of women to medical studies from the twelfth to the fourteenth centuries was not only not discouraged, but was distinctly encouraged, and we find evidence that a number of women studied and taught medicine, wrote books on medical subjects, were consulted with regard to medico-legal questions, and in general were looked upon as medical colleagues in practically every sense of the word. The very first medical school that developed in modern times, that of Salerno, which came into European prominence in the eleventh century, was quite early in its history opened to women students, and a number of women professors were on its faculty.

Considering the modern idea that ours is the first time when women have ever had any real opportunity for the higher education, and above all professional education, it is a source of no little astonishment to find that at Salerno not only an opportunity was afforded to women to study medicine, but the department of women's diseases was handed over entirely to them, and as a consequence we have a Salernitan School of Women Physicians, some of whom wrote textbooks on the subject relating to this speciality. De Renzi, in his "Storia della Scuola di Salerno," has brought to light many details of the history of this phase of medical education for women at the first important medical school that developed in modern Europe. The best known of these medieval women physicians was Trotula, to whom is attributed a series of books on medical subjects—though doubtless some of these were due rather to disciples, but became identified with the more famous master, as so often happened with medieval books. Trotula's most important book bears two sub-titles: "Trotula's Unique Book for the Curing of Diseases of Women, Before, During, and After Labour," and the other sub-title, "Trotula's Wonderful Book of Experiences (*experimentalis*) in the Diseases of

Women, Before, During, and After Labour, with Other Details Likewise Relating to Labour."

Probably the most interesting passage in her book for the modern time is that with regard to a torn perineum and its repair, even when prolapse of the uterus is a complication. The passage, which may be found readily in De Renzi or in Gurlt, runs:

"Certain patients, from the severity of the labour, run into a rupture of the genitalia. In some even the vulva and anus become one foramen, having the same course. As a consequence, prolapse of the uterus occurs, and it becomes indurated. In order to relieve this condition, we apply to the uterus warm wine in which butter has been boiled, and these fomentations are continued until the uterus becomes soft, and then it is gently replaced. After this we sew the tear between the anus and vulva in three or four places with silk thread. The woman should then be placed in bed, with the feet elevated, and must retain that position, even for eating and drinking, and all the necessities of life, for eight or nine days. During this time, also, there must be no bathing, and care must be taken to avoid everything that might cause coughing, and all indigestible materials."

There is a passage almost more interesting with regard to prophylaxis of rupture of the perineum. Trotula says: "In order to avoid the aforesaid danger, careful provision should be made, and precautions should be taken during labour after the following fashion: A cloth folded in somewhat oblong shape should be placed on the anus, and during every effort for the expulsion of the child, that should be pressed firmly, in order that there may not be any solution of the continuity of tissue."

There are records of other women professors of Salerno, though none of them as famous as Trotula. A lady of the name of Mercuriade is said to have written "On Crises in Pestilent Fever," and as she occupied herself with surgery as well as medicine, there is also a work on "The Cure of Wounds." Rebecca Guarna, who belonged to the old Salernitan family of that name, a member of which in the twelfth century was Romuald, priest, physician, and historian, wrote "On Fevers," "On the Urine," and "On the Embryo." Abella acquired a great reputation with her work "On Black Bile," and curiously enough on "The Nature of Seminal Fluid." From these books it is clear that, while as professors they had charge of the department of women's diseases, they studied all branches of medicine. There are a number of licences preserved in the Archives of Naples in which women are accorded the privilege of practising medicine, and apparently these licences were without limitation as to the scope of practice. The preamble of the licence, however, suggests the eminent suitability of women treating women's diseases. It ran as follows:

"Since, then, the law permits women to exercise the profession of physicians, and since, besides, due regard being had to purity of morals, women are better suited for the treatment of women's diseases, after having received the oath of fidelity, we permit," etc.

The story of medical education for women with the free opportunity for practice, and above all the recognition accorded by making them professors at the University of Salerno, will seem all the more surprising to those who recall that the Benedictines largely influenced the foundation at Salerno, and were important factors in its subsequent growth and management. Ordinarily it would be presumed that monastic influence would be distinctly against permitting women to secure such opportunities for education, and, above all, encouraging their occupation with medical practice. As a matter of fact, it seems indeed to have been monastic influence which secured this special development. The Benedictines were already habituated to the idea that women were quite capable, if given the opportunity, of taking advantage of the highest education; and besides, they were accustomed to see them occupied, and successfully, with the care of the ailing. When St. Benedict established the monks of the West in retreats, where the men of the earlier Middle Ages could secure, in the midst of troubled times and with men in the cities utterly neglectful of intellectual interests, a refuge from the disturbed life around them, and an opportunity for intellectual development, his sister Scholastica afforded similar opportunities for such women as felt that they were called rather to the intellectual and spiritual life than to the taking up of the burden of domestic duties and a wife's labours.

In these Benedictine convents for women, as they spread throughout Italy—and afterwards throughout Germany, and France, and England, though the fact is often ignored—the intellectual life was pursued as faithfully as the spiritual. Besides, there gathered around the convent gates as around the monasteries the farmers who worked their estates, and who found it so good "to live under the crozier," as the rule of the Abbot or Abbess was called, and who always suffered severely whenever, by confiscation or war or like disturbances, the monastic lands passed into the hands of laymen. For their own large numbers as well as for their peasantry, and for the travellers who stayed in their guest-houses, the nuns had to provide medical attendance; and the infirmarians of the convents, situated as they were so often far from cities or towns, acquired considerable medical knowledge and came to apply it with excellent success. The traditions were gathered from many quarters, and passed on for centuries from one house to another; and they gathered simples and treated the ordinary ailments, and nursed the ailing into moods of greater courage and states of mind that predisposed to recovery.

Probably the most important book on medicine that we have from the twelfth century is written by a Benedictine Abbess, since known as St. Hildegarde. She was born of noble parents at Boeckelheim in the county of Sponheim, about the end of the eleventh century. She was educated at the Benedictine cloister of Disibodenberg, and when her education was finished she entered the house as a religious, and at the age of about fifty she became abbess. Her writings, reputation for sanctity, and her wise rule, eminently sympathetic as she was, attracted so many new members to the community that the convent became overcrowded. Accordingly, with eighteen of her nuns, Hildegarde withdrew to a new convent at Rupertsburg, which English and American travellers will doubtless recall because it is not far from Bingen on the Rhine, made famous in the later time by Mrs. Hemans's poem. Here she came to be a sort of centre for the intellectual life of her period. According to traditions, some of which are dubious, she was in active correspondence with nearly every important personage of her generation. She was an intimate friend of St. Bernard of Clairvaux, who was himself perhaps the most influential man of Europe in this century. Her correspondence was enormous, and she was consulted from all sides because her advice on difficult problems of any and every kind was considered so valuable.

In spite of all this time-taking correspondence she found leisure to write a series of books, most of them on mystical subjects, but two of them, strange as it may seem, on medicine. The first is called "Liber Simplicis Medicinæ," and the second "Liber Compositæ Medicinæ." These books were written as a contribution of her views with regard to the medical knowledge of her time, but were evidently due, partly at least, to the Benedictine traditions of interest in medicine. Dr. Melanie Lipinska in her "Histoire des Femmes Médicins," a thesis presented for the doctorate in medicine at the University of Paris in 1900, which was subsequently awarded a special prize by the French Academy, reviews Hildegarde's work critically from the medical standpoint. She does not hesitate to declare the Abbess Hildegarde the most important medical writer of her time. Reuss, the editor of the works of Hildegarde as they are published in Migne's "Patrologia," the immense French edition of all the important works of the Fathers, Doctors, and Saints of the Church, says:

"Among all the saintly religious who have practised medicine or written about it in the Middle Ages, the most important is without any doubt St. Hildegarde...." With regard to her book he says: "All those who wish to write the history of the medical and natural sciences must read this work, in which this religious woman, evidently well grounded in all that was known at that time in the secrets of nature, discusses and examines carefully all the knowledge of the time." He adds: "It is certain that St. Hildegarde knew many things that were unknown to the physicians of her time."

Some of Hildegarde's expressions are startling enough because they indicate discussion of, and attempts to elucidate, problems which many people of the modern time are likely to think occurred only to the last few generations. For instance, in talking about the stars and describing their course through the firmament, she makes use of a comparison that seems strangely ahead of her time. She says: "Just as the blood moves in the veins, causing them to vibrate and pulsate, so the stars move in the firmament, and send out sparks as it were of light, like the vibrations of the veins." This is, of course, not an anticipation of the discovery of the circulation of the blood, but it shows how close were men's ideas to some such thought five centuries before Harvey's discovery. For Hildegarde the brain was the regulator of all the vital qualities, the centre of life. She connects the nerves in their passage from the brain and the spinal cord through the body with manifestations of life. She has a series of chapters with regard to psychology, normal and morbid. She talks about frenzy, insanity, despair, dread, obsession, anger, idiocy, and innocency. She says very strongly in one place that "when headache and migraine and vertigo attack a patient simultaneously, they render a man foolish and upset his reason. This makes many people think that he is possessed of a demon, but that is not true." These are the exact words of the saint as quoted in Mlle. Lipinska's thesis.

With this story of St. Hildegarde in mind, and the recall of other educational developments among the Benedictine nuns, it is easy to understand the developments that took place at Salerno, where monastic influence was so prominent. Just as the medical, and above all the surgical, traditions of Salerno found their way to Bologna at the beginning of the thirteenth century, so also did the regulations regarding standards in medical education, and with them medical education for women. There are definite historical documents which show that women not only studied but taught in the medical department of Bologna. The name of one of them at least is very well known. She was Alessandra Giliani, and, strange as it might appear, was one of the prosectors in anatomy of Mondino, the founder of teaching by human dissection. According to the "Cronaca Persicetana," quoted by Medici in his "History of the Anatomical School at Bologna":

"She became most valuable to Mondino because she would cleanse most skilfully the smallest vein, the arteries, all ramifications of the vessels, without lacerating or dividing them, and to prepare them for demonstration she would fill them with various coloured liquids, which, after having been driven into the vessels, would harden without destroying the vessels. Again, she would paint these same vessels to their minute branches so perfectly, and colour them so naturally, that, added to the wonderful explanations and teachings of the master, they brought him great fame and credit."

This passage with its description, as coming from a woman, of a very early anticipation of our most modern anatomical technique—injection, hardening, and colouring, so as to imitate nature for the making of anatomical preparations, for class and demonstration purposes—is all the more interesting because the next great improvement in anatomical teaching, the use of wax models of dissected specimens coloured to imitate nature, came also from a woman, Madame Manzolini, also of Bologna. Feminine instinct aroused women to use their inventive ability to do away with the necessity for always recurring to the deterrent material of fresh dissections, and yet securing such preparations as would make teaching not less but more effective.

Some doubt has been thrown on certain details of the story of Alessandra Giliani, but the memorial tablet erected at the time of her death in the Hospital Church of Santa Maria de Mareto in Florence gives all the important facts, and tells the story of the grief of her fiancé, who was himself Mondino's other assistant. Like her, he died young also, when there were high hopes of his ability, and there is more than the suspicion that these two untimely deaths may have been due to dissecting wound infections. She died "consumed by her labours," so that it may have been phthisis; but he was taken by "a swift and lamentable death."

Nicaise, in the Introduction to his edition of Guy de Chauliac's "Grande Chirurgie" (Paris, 1893), has a brief review of the history of women in medicine, with special reference to France. He supplies practically all the information available in very short compass, as well as the references where more details can be obtained.

"Women continued to practise medicine in Italy for centuries, and the names of some who attained great renown have been preserved for us. Their works are still quoted from in the fifteenth century.

"There was none of them in France who became distinguished, but women could practise medicine in certain towns at least on condition of passing an examination before regularly appointed masters. An edict of 1311, at the same time that it interdicts unauthorized women from practising surgery, recognizes their rights to practise the art if they have undergone an examination before the regularly appointed master surgeons of the corporation of Paris. An edict of King John, April, 1352, contains the same expressions as the previous edict. Du Bouley, in his 'History of the University of Paris' gives another edict by the same king, also published in the year 1352, as a result of the complaints of the faculties at Paris, in which there is also question of women physicians. This responded to a petition: 'Having heard the petition of the Dean and Masters of the Faculty of Medicine at the University of Paris, who declare that there are very many of both sexes, some of the women with legal title to practise and some of them merely old pretenders to a knowledge of medicine, who come to Paris in order to practise, be it enacted,' etc. (The edict then proceeds to repeat the terms of previous legislation in this matter.)

"Guy de Chauliac speaks also of women who practised surgery. They formed the fifth and last class of operators in his time. He complains that they are accustomed to too great an extent to give over patients suffering from all kinds of maladies to the will of Heaven, founding their practice on the maxim, 'The Lord has given as he has pleased; the Lord will take away when he pleases; may the name of the Lord be blessed.'

"In the sixteenth century, according to Pasquier, the practice of medicine by women almost entirely disappeared. The number of women physicians becomes more and more rare in the following centuries, just in proportion as we approach our own time. Pasquier says that we find a certain number of them anxious for knowledge, and with a special penchant for the study of the natural sciences and even of medicine, but very few of them take up practice."

There seems, however, to have been not nearly so much freedom or so much encouragement for women in medicine in France as in Italy. Indeed, in the whole matter of education for women, medieval France has but little to record compared to Italy's significant chapter in the history of feminine education. One reason for this was doubtless the Héloïse-Abélard incident early in the history of the University of Paris. This seems to have discouraged efforts in the direction of the securing of the higher education for women in most of the Western Universities. Oxford was a daughter university of Paris, and Cambridge of Oxford, and they and all the other universities of the West were more deeply influenced in their customs and organization by Paris than by Italy, and as a consequence we hear little of feminine education in the West generally. One result of this has been the existence of a feeling that, since women had very few opportunities for the higher education in Western Europe, they must have had them nowhere else. This presumption forms the basis of not a little misunderstanding of the Middle Ages in our time. It often takes but a little incident to set the current of history in a very different direction from that in which it might have gone, and this seems to have been the case as regards the higher education for women in France and Spain and England.

CHAPTER X

MEDIEVAL HOSPITALS

Our recent experience makes it easy to understand that such magnificent advance in surgery as has been described in the preceding chapters would have been quite impossible unless there were excellent hospitals in the medieval period. Good surgery demands good hospitals, and indeed inevitably creates them. Whenever hospitals are in a state of neglect, surgery is hopeless. We have, however, abundant evidence of the existence of fine hospitals in the Middle Ages, quite apart from this assumption of them, because of the surprising surgery of the period. Historical traditions from the earlier as well as the later medieval times demonstrate a magnificent development of hospital organization. While there had been military hospitals and a few civic institutions for the care of citizens in Roman times, and some hospital traditions in the East and in connection with the temples in Egypt, hospital organization as we know it is Christian in origin; and particularly the erection of institutions for the care of the ailing poor came to be looked upon very early as a special duty of Christians. Even the Roman Emperor, Julian the Apostate, declared that the old Olympian religion would inevitably lose its hold on the people, unless somehow it could show such care for others in need as the Christians exhibited wherever they obtained a foothold. It was not, however, until nearly the beginning of the Middle Ages that the Christians were in sufficient numbers in the cities, and were free enough from interference by government, to take up seriously the problem of public hospital organization. The rapidity of the development, once external obstacles were removed, shows clearly how close to the heart of Christianity was the subject of care for the ailing poor. St. Basil's magnificent foundation at Cæsarea in Cappadocia, called the *Basilias*, which took on the dimensions of a city (termed Newtown) with regular streets, buildings for different classes of patients, dwellings for physicians and nurses and for the convalescent, and apparently even workshops and industrial schools for the care and instruction of foundlings and of children that had been under the care of the monastery, as well as for what we would now call reconstruction work, shows how far hospital organization, even in the latter part of the fourth century, had developed.

About the year 400 Fabiola at Rome, according to St. Jerome, "established a Nosocomium to gather in the sick from the streets, and to nurse the wretched sufferers wasted from poverty and disease." A little later Pammachius, a Roman Senator, founded a Xenodochium for the care of strangers which St. Jerome praises in one of his letters. At the end of the fifth century Pope Symmachus built hospitals in connection with the three most important churches of Rome, St. Peter's, St. Paul's, and St. Lawrence's. During the Pontificate of Vigilius, Belisarius founded a Xenodochium in the *Via Lata* at Rome, shortly after the middle of the sixth century. Christian hospitals were early established in the cities of France; and not long after the conversion of England, in that country.

In connection with these hospitals, it is rather easy to understand the fine development of surgery by early Christian physicians which we have traced. The later medieval period of hospital building, however, is of particular interest in the history of medicine, because we have such details of it as show its excellent adaptation to medical and surgical needs. According to Virchow, in his article on the History of German Hospitals, which is to be found in the second volume of his collected "Essays on Public Medicine and the History of Epidemics,"[14] the story of the foundation of these hospitals of the Middle Ages, even those of Germany, centres around the name of one man, Pope Innocent III. Virchow was not at all a papistically inclined writer, so that his tribute to the great Pope who solved so finely the medico-social problems of his time undoubtedly represents a merited recognition of a great social development in history.

"The beginning of the history of all these German hospitals is connected with the name of that Pope who made the boldest and farthest-reaching attempt to gather the sum of human interests into the organization of the Catholic Church. The hospitals of the Holy Ghost were one of the many means by which Innocent III. thought to hold humanity to the Holy See. And surely it was one of the most effective. Was it not calculated to create the most profound impression to see how the mighty Pope, who humbled emperors and deposed kings, who was the unrelenting adversary of the Albigenses, turned his eyes sympathetically upon the poor and the sick, sought the helpless and the neglected upon the streets, and saved the illegitimate children from death in the waters! There is something at once conciliating and fascinating in the fact that, at the very time when the fourth crusade was inaugurated through his influence, the thought of founding a great organization of an essentially humane character, which was eventually to extend throughout all Christendom, was also taking form in his soul; and that in the same year (1204) in which the new Latin Empire was founded in Constantinople, the newly erected hospital of the Holy Spirit, by the old bridge on the other side of the Tiber, was blessed and dedicated as the future centre of this organization."

According to tradition, just about the beginning of the thirteenth century Pope Innocent resolved to build a hospital in Rome. On inquiry, he found that probably the best man to put in charge of hospital organization was Guy or Guido of Montpellier, of the Brothers of the Holy Ghost, who had founded a hospital at

Montpellier which became famous throughout Europe for its thorough organization. Accordingly he summoned Guido to Rome, and gave into his hands the organization of the new hospital, which was erected on the other side of Tiber in the Borgo not far from St. Peter's. Indeed, Santo Spirito Hospital, as it came to be called, was probably the direct successor of the hospital which Pope Symmachus (488-514) had had built in connection with St. Peter's not long after the beginning of the Middle Ages. It is easy to understand that at the time when magnificent municipal structures, cathedrals, town halls, abbeys, and educational institutions of various kinds were being erected, with exemplary devotion to art and use, the Hospital of Santo Spirito under the special patronage of the Pope was not unworthy of its time.[15] We know very little, however, about the actual structure.

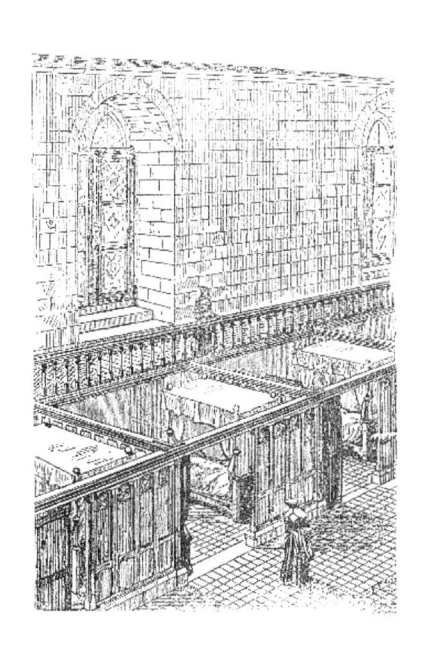

THIRTEENTH-CENTURY HOSPITAL INTERIOR (TONERRE)
From "The Thirteenth: Greatest of Centuries," by J. J. Walsh

Then, as now, Bishops made regular visits at intervals *ad limina*—that is, to the Pope as Chief Bishop of the Church; and according to tradition Pope Innocent called their attention particularly to this hospital of Santo Spirito, one of his favourite institutions, and suggested that every diocese in Christendom ought to have such a refuge for the ailing poor. The consequence was the erection of hospitals everywhere throughout Europe. Virchow has told the story of these hospital foundations of the Holy Ghost, as they were called, and makes it very clear that probably every town of 5,000 inhabitants everywhere throughout Europe at this time had a hospital. The traditions with regard to France are quite as complete as those that concern Germany and the great hospitals of London—St. Thomas's; St. Bartholomew's, which had been a priory with a house for the care of the poor, but was now turned into a hospital; Bethlehem, afterwards Bedlam; Bridewell, and Christ's Hospital, the first of which afterwards became a prison, while Christ's Hospital, though retaining its name, became a school. The Five Royal Hospitals, as they were called, were either founded, or received a great stimulus and thorough reorganization, during the thirteenth century.

It would be easy to suppose these hospitals were rather rude structures, inexpertly built, poorly arranged, and above all badly lighted and ventilated. They might be expected to furnish protection from the elements for the poor, but scarcely more, and probably became in the course of time hotbeds of infection because of their lack of air and uncleanness. As a matter of fact, they were almost exactly the opposite of any such supposition. Those in the larger towns at least were model hospitals in many ways, and ever so much better than many hospital structures erected in post-medieval centuries. Indeed, the ordinary impression as to the medieval hospitals, and their lack of suitability to their purpose, would apply perfectly to the hospitals of the latter half of the eighteenth and the early nineteenth centuries. It is because our generation still has the memory of these hospitals of the past generation, and assumes that if these were so bad, the hospitals of an earlier time must have been worse and the hospitals of the medieval period must have been intolerable, that the derogatory tradition with regard to medieval hospitals and many other medical subjects maintained itself until the coming of real information with regard to them.

The ecclesiastical architecture of the later Middle Ages was not only beautiful, but it was eminently suitable for its purpose, and above all provided light and air. The churches, the town halls, the monasteries and abbeys, were models in their kind, and it would have been quite surprising if the hospitals alone had been unworthy products of that great architectural period. As abundant remains serve to show even to the present time, they were not. The hospitals built in the thirteenth century particularly usually were of one story, had high ceilings with large windows, often were built near the water in order that there might be abundance of water for cleansing purposes, and also so that the sewage of the hospital might be carried off, had tiled floors that facilitated thorough cleansing, and many other provisions that the architects of our time are reintroducing into hospital construction. They were a complete contrast to the barrack-like hospitals with small windows, narrow corridors, cell-like rooms, which were built even two generations ago, and which represented the lowest period in hospital building for seven centuries.

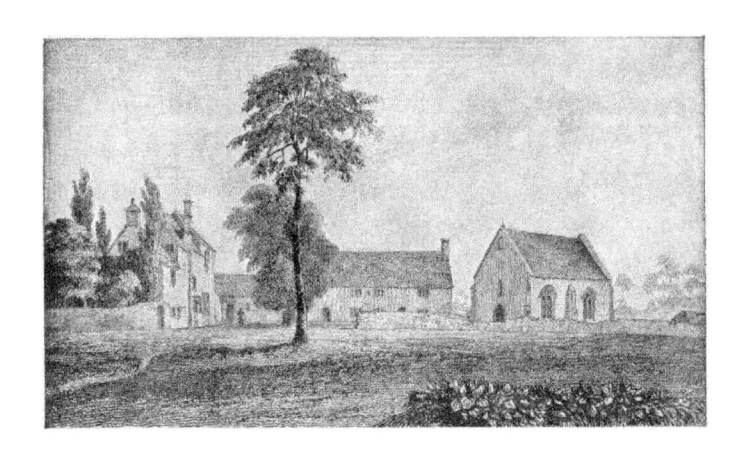

LEPER HOSPITAL OF ST. BARTHOLOMEW, OXFORD
From "Medieval Hospitals," by Miss R. M. Clay

Viollet le Duc, in his "Dictionary of Architecture," has given a picture of the interior of one of these medieval hospitals, that of Tonnerre in France, erected by Marguerite of Bourgogne, the sister of St. Louis, in 1293, which we reproduce here. Mr. Arthur Dillon, discussing this hospital from the standpoint of an architect, says:

"It was an admirable hospital in every way, and it is doubtful if we to-day surpass it. It was isolated, the ward was separated from the other buildings, it had the advantages we so often lose of being but one story high, and more space was given to each patient than we can now afford.

"The ventilation by the great windows and ventilators in the ceiling was excellent; it was cheerfully lighted, and the arrangement of the gallery shielded the patients from dazzling light and from draughts from the windows, and afforded an easy means of supervision; while the division by the roofless, low partitions isolated the sick, and obviated the depression that comes from the sight of others in pain.

"It was, moreover, in great contrast to the cheerless white wards of to-day. The vaulted ceiling was very beautiful; the woodwork was richly carved, and the great windows over the altars were filled with coloured glass. Altogether, it was one of the best examples of the best period of Gothic architecture."

The hospital ward itself was 55 feet wide and 270 feet long and had a high arched ceiling of wood. The Princess herself lived in a separate building, connected with the hospital by a covered passage. The kitchen and storehouse for provisions were also in separate buildings. The whole hospital plant was placed between the branches of a small stream conducted around it, which served to temper the atmosphere, and was a source of water supply at one end of the grounds and helped in the disposal of sewage from the other end.

A hospital of the Holy Ghost which may be taken as the type of such structures is still standing at Lübeck in Germany, and was, like the hospital at Tonnerre, also built during the thirteenth century. It was erected as the result of the movement initiated by Pope Innocent's foundation of the Santo Spirito at Rome. The picture of this, in my "Thirteenth Century," will serve to show what Holy Ghost hospitals in important cities at least were like. Lübeck was one of the rich Hansa towns in the thirteenth century, but there were many others of equal importance, or very nearly so, and all of these towns were rivals in the architectural adornment of their municipalities, and particularly in the erection of cathedrals, town halls, guild halls, and other buildings for the use of citizens.

The older portion of the Hospital of St. Jean at Bruges also gives an excellent idea of a later medieval hospital as it was constructed in a populous commercial town. Bruges, almost needless to say, was one of the most important cities of Europe in the fourteenth century. The Hospital of St. Jean, then, was built, like the cathedral and churches and the town hall, so as to be worthy of the city's prestige. The older part, which is now used for a storeroom, has the characteristics of the best medieval hospitals. The ward was one story in height, the windows were large, high in the walls, and the canals that flowed around the hospital made pleasant vistas for the patient, while the gardens attached were eminently suitable for convalescents. The phases of hospital building down the centuries can be studied at St. Jean, and, strange as it may seem, the oldest portion of the hospital, that of the medieval period, provided the most light and air for the patients and the best opportunity for thorough cleansing, as well as for occupation of the patients' minds with details of the construction that were visible from any part of the ward. The hospitals of the Middle Ages are particularly interesting, because they represent a solution of the social problems other than merely the relief of pain and suffering, or the care of the needy who have none to care for them. They represent a ready, constantly near opportunity for the better-to-do classes to exercise charity toward those who needed it most. The hospitals were always in the busiest portions of the towns, and were often visited by the citizens, both men and women. Dr. John S. Billings, in his description of "The Johns Hopkins Hospital" (Baltimore, 1890), touched upon this spirit of the hospital movement of the Middle Ages in a very appropriate way when he said:

"When the medieval priest established in each great city of France a Hotel Dieu, a place for God's hospitality, it was in the interest of charity as he understood it, including both the helping of the sick poor, and the affording of those who were neither sick nor poor an opportunity and a stimulus to help their fellow-men; and doubtless the cause of humanity and religion was advanced more by the effect on the givers than on the receivers."

A rather significant historical detail with regard to medieval hospitals is the foundation of a special order to take care of the hospitals in which St. Anthony's Fire, or what we know as erysipelas, was treated. Apparently this indicated the recognition of the contagiousness of this disease by the medieval people. Pope Honorius III. approved the foundation of an order of nurses particularly devoted to the care of patients suffering from this affection. Other religious congregations for the same works seem to have been established. We did not recognize the contagiousness of the disease until the last generation. Undoubtedly these special foundations made it possible to control many of the epidemics of erysipelas that used to make surgical care in our hospitals in the modern time such a difficult matter. Even as late as our Civil War here in America, erysipelas was the special dread of the hospital surgeon. Oliver Wendell Holmes pointed out that erysipelas might readily be carried to the parturient woman with the production of child-bed fever. It is interesting to realize, then, the attempt of the medieval period to segregate the disease.

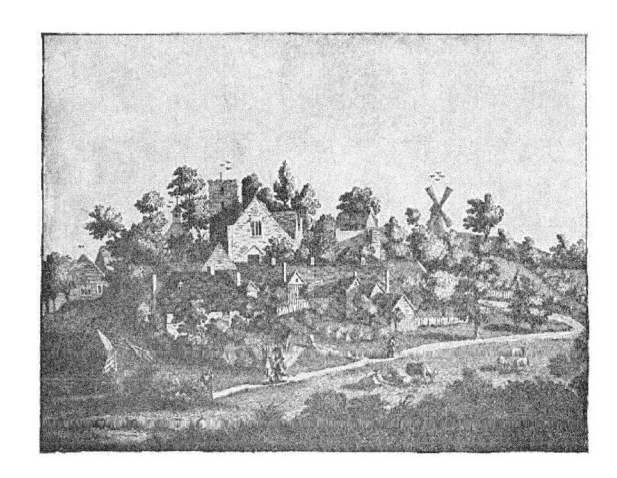

THE HARBLEDOWN HOSPITAL, NEAR CANTERBURY
From "Medieval Hospitals," by Miss R. M. Clay

"On the outskirts of a town, seven hundred years ago, the eye of the traveller would have been caught by a well-known landmark—a group of cottages, with an adjoining chapel, clustering round a green enclosure. At a glance he would recognize it as the lazar-house, and would prepare to throw an alms to the crippled and disfigured representative of the community."]

Besides hospitals, a series of lazarettos—that is, of buildings for the segregation of lepers—were erected in the various countries of Europe during the medieval period. Just about the end of the Crusades it was discovered that leprosy had become very common throughout Europe. It is often said that leprosy was introduced at this time, but it had evidently been in the West for many centuries before. Gregory of Tours mentions leper hospitals as early as 560, and the disease evidently continued to progress, in spite of these special hospitals, until in the thirteenth century it became clear that strenuous efforts would have to be made to wipe out the disease. Accordingly, leproseries were erected in connection with practically every town in Europe at this time. Baas estimates that there were some 19,000 of them in Europe altogether. Virchow has listed a large number of the leper hospitals of the German cities, quite enough to show that probably no organized community was without one.

As a consequence of this widespread movement of enforced segregation, leprosy gradually died out in Europe, remaining only here and there in backward localities. The disease was probably as common during the later Middle Ages as tuberculosis is among us at the present time. The recently discovered relations between the bacterial cause of the two diseases may give rise to the question as to whether we shall succeed as well with the great social and hygienic problem that confronts our generation, of lowering the death-rate from "the great white plague," as the medieval generations did with their chronic folk-disease, leprosy. It would be "a consummation devoutly to be wished." We are now beginning to have as many sanatoria for tuberculosis in proportion to the population as they had of leproseries. These leproseries, or lazarettos, as they were called, were not at all the dreadful places that the imagination has been wont to picture them in recent years; on the contrary they were, as a rule, beautifully situated on a side-hill to favour drainage, consisted of a series of dwellings with a chapel in their midst surrounded by trees, and encompassed by what was altogether a park effect. Miss Clay, in "Medieval Hospitals," has given a picture of one of them, which we reproduce, because it serves to contradict the popular false notion with regard to the bare and ugly and more or less jail-like character of these institutions.

CHAPTER XI
MEDIEVAL CARE OF THE INSANE

Quite contrary to the usual impression, rather extensive and well-managed institutions for the care of the insane came into existence during the Middle Ages, and continued to fulfil a very necessary social and medical duty. For the unspeakable neglect of the insane which is a disgrace to civilization, we must look to the centuries much nearer our own than those of the Middle Ages. Above all, the Middle Ages did not segregate the insane entirely from other ailing patients until their affections had become so chronic as to be certainly incurable, and they took the insane into ordinary hospitals to care for them at the beginning of their affection. This mode of procedure has many advantages, mainly in getting the patients out of unfavourable environments and putting them under skilled care early in their affections, so that a definite effort is being made to restore what is called the psychopathic ward in the general hospitals in our time. Only a careful study of the details of actual historical references to the medieval care of the insane will serve to contradict unfortunate traditions which have gathered around the subject entirely without justification in real history.

The traditions of medical knowledge with regard to the insane inherited by the early Middle Ages from the ancients were of the best, and the books written at this time have some interesting material on the subject. Paulus Aëgineta (Aëginetus), who wrote in the seventh century—and it must not be forgotten that already at this time some 200 years of the Middle Ages have passed—has some excellent directions with regard to the care and treatment of patients suffering from melancholia and mania. He says, in his paragraph on the cure of melancholy: "Those who are subject to melancholy from a primary affection of the brain are to be treated with frequent baths and a wholesome and humid diet, together with suitable exhilaration of mind, and without any other remedy unless, when from its long continuance, the offending humour is difficult to evacuate, in which case we must have recourse to more powerful and complicated plans of treatment." He then gives a series of directions, some of them quite absurd to us, apparently in order to satisfy those who feel that they must keep on doing something for these cases, though evidently his own opinion is expressed in the first portion of the paragraph, and in the simple laxative treatment that he outlines. "These cases are to be purged first with dodder of thyme (*epithymus*) or aloes; for if a small quantity of these be taken every day it will be of the greatest service, and open the bowels gently."

His directions as to diet for those suffering from melancholia are all in the line of limiting the consumption of materials that might possibly cause digestive disturbance, for evidently his experience had taught him that the depression was deeper whenever indigestion occurs. He says: "The diet for melancholics shall be wholesome and moderately moistening; abstaining from beef, roe's flesh, dried lentils, cabbages, snails, thick and dark coloured wines, and in a word from whatever things engender black bile." Mania was to be treated very nearly like melancholia, with special warnings as to the necessity for particular care of these patients. "But above all things they must be secured in bed, so that they may not be able to injure themselves or those who approach them; or swung within a wicker basket in a small couch suspended from on high." This last suggestion would seem to be eminently practical, especially for young people who are not too heavy, and enforces the idea that the physicians of this time were thinking seriously of their problems of care for the insane and exercising their ingenuity in inventions for their benefit.

Paul of Ægina seems, then, to have thought that mania and melancholia were definitely related to each other, and to have held a similar opinion in this regard to Aretæus, who declared that melancholia was an incipient mania. Both had evidently noted that in most cases there were melancholic and maniacal stages in the same patient. These early medieval students of mental disease, then, anticipated to a rather startling extent our most recent conclusions with regard to the essential insanities. They would have been much readier to agree with Kraepelin's term, manic-depressive insanity, than with the teaching of the hundred years before our time, which so absolutely separated these two conditions.

All this represents an organized knowledge of insanity that could not be acquired by chance, nor by a few intermittent observations on a small number of patients, but must have been due to actual, careful, continued observation of many of them over a long period. Here is the presumptive evidence for the existence of special institutions for their care at this period in the Middle Ages. This presumption is confirmed by Ducange in his "Commentary on Byzantine History," in which he tells of the existence of a *morotrophium*, or house for lunatics, at Byzantium in the fourth century, and one is known to have existed at Jerusalem late in the fifth century. Further confirmation of the existence of special arrangements and institutions for the care of the insane even thus early in the Middle Ages is obtained from the *regula monachorum* of St. Jerome, which enjoins upon the monks the duty of making careful provision for the isolation and proper treatment of the sick both in mind and body, whilst they were enjoined to leave nothing undone to secure appropriate care and speedy recovery of such patients.[16]

Among the first Christian institutions for the care of the ailing founded by private benevolence, a refuge for the insane was undoubtedly built in England before the seventh century. Burdett says that: "How far the two institutions established in England prior to A.D. 700 were entitled to be considered asylums, we have discovered insufficient evidence to enable us to decide." He evidently inclines to the opinion, however, that provision was made in them for the care of those ailing in mind as well as in body.

There is a rather well-grounded tradition that Sigibaldus, the thirty-sixth bishop of Metz during the papacy of Leo IV., about A.D. 850, erected two monasteries and paid special attention to the sick in body and mind. There are records that the insane in Metz were placed under the guardianship of persons regularly appointed. The attendants in the hospitals had to take a special oath of allegiance to the King, and that they would fulfil their duties properly.

There is definite evidence of Bethlehem in London, afterwards known as Bedlam, containing lunatics during the thirteenth century, for there is the report of a Royal Commission in the next century stating that there were six lunatics there who were under duress. Burdett says that Bedlam has been devoted exclusively to the treatment of lunatics from some years prior to 1400 down to the present time, so that it takes precedence in this matter of the asylum founded in Valencia in Spain, which Desmaisons has erroneously held as the first established in Europe. Esquirol states that the Parliament of Paris ordered the general hospital, that of the Hotel Dieu, to provide a place for the confinement of lunatics centuries before this; and while definite evidence is lacking, there seems no doubt that in most places there were, as we have said, what we would call psychopathic wards in connection with medieval hospitals.

Early in the fifteenth century there are a number of bequests made to Bedlam which specifically mention the care of the insane. Indeed, "the poor madmen of Bethlehem" seem to have been favourite objects of charity. The care of the insane there seems to have touched a responsive chord in many hearts. Mayor Gregory describes in his "Historical Collections" (about 1451) this London asylum and its work of mercy, and from him we have evidence of the fact that some of the patients were restored to reason after their stay in the asylum. He has words of praise for how "honestly" the patients were cared for; but recognizes, of course, that some could not be cured. In his quaint old English he emphasizes particularly the church feature of the establishment.

"A chyrche of Owre Lady that ys namyde Bedlam. And yn that place ben founde many men that ben fallyn owte of hyr wytte. And fulle honestely they ben kepte in that place; and sum ben restoryde unto hyr witte and helthe a-gayne. And sum ben a-bydyng there yn for evyr, for they ben falle soo moche owte of hem selfe that hyt ys uncurerabylle unto man."

In her chapter on Hospitals for the Insane in "Medieval Hospitals of England,"[17] Miss Clay gives a number of details of the care of the insane in England, and notes that the Rolls of Parliament (1414) mention "hospitals ... to maintain men and women who had lost their wits and memory"; manifestly they had some experience which differentiated cases of aphasia from those of insanity. She says that outside of London "it was customary to receive persons suffering from attacks of mania into general infirmaries. At Holy Trinity, Salisbury, not only were sick persons and women in childbirth received, but mad people were to be taken care of (*furiosi custodiantur donec sensum adipiscantur*). This was at the close of the fourteenth century. In the petition for the reformation of hospitals (1414), it is stated that they existed partly to maintain those who had lost their wits and memory (*hors de leur sennes et mémoire*)."

Further evidence of the presence of the insane with other patients is to be found in the fact that in certain hospitals and almshouses it was forbidden to receive the insane, showing that in many places that must have been the custom. Miss Clay notes:

"Many almshouse-statutes, however, prohibited their admission. A regulation concerning an endowed bed in St. John's, Coventry (1444), declared that a candidate must be 'not mad, quarrelsome, leprous, infected.' At Ewelme 'no wood man' [crazy person] must be received; and an inmate becoming 'madd, or woode,' was to be removed from the Croydon almshouse."

Desmaisons is responsible for the tradition which declares there were no asylums for the insane until the beginning of the fifteenth century, and that then they were founded by the Spaniards under the influence of the Mohammedans. Lecky, in his "History of European Morals," has contradicted this assertion of Desmaisons', and declares that there is absolutely no proof for it. Burdett, in his "History of Hospitals," vol. i., p. 42, says with regard to this question:

"Again, Desmaisons states that the 'origin of the first establishment exclusively devoted to the insane dates back to A.D. 1409. This date constitutes an historic fact, the importance of which doubtless needs no demonstration. Its importance stands out all the more clearly when we calculate the lapse of time between the period just spoken of (1409) and that in which Spain's example' (Desmaisons is here referring to the Valencia asylum as the first in Europe) 'found so many followers.' Now, as a matter of fact, an asylum exclusively for the use of the mentally infirm existed at Metz in the year A.D. 1100, and another at Elbing, near Danzic, in 1320. Again, there was an ancient asylum, according to Dugdale, known as Berking Church Hospital, near the Tower of London, for which Robert Denton, chaplain, obtained a licence from King Edward III. in A.D. 1371. Denton paid forty shillings for this licence, which empowered him to found a hospital in a house of his own, in the parish of Berking Church, London, 'for the poor priests, and for men and women in the said city who suddenly fall into a frenzy and lose their memory, who were to reside there till cured; with an oratory to the said hospital to the invocation of the Blessed Virgin Mary.'"

The passages from Aëgineta at the beginning of this chapter represent a thorough understanding of mental diseases often supposed not to exist at this time. Often it is presumed that this thorough appreciation of insanity gradually disappeared during subsequent centuries, and was not revived until almost our own time. It is quite easy, however, to illustrate by quotations from the second half of the Middle Ages a like sensible treatment of the subject of insanity by scientific and even popular writers. How different was the attitude of mind of the medieval people toward lunacy from that which is usually assumed as existing at that time may be gathered very readily from the paragraph in "Bartholomeus' Encyclopædia" with regard to madness. I doubt whether in a brief discussion so much that is absolutely true could be better said in our time. Insanity, according to old Bartholomew, was due to some poison, autointoxication, or strong drink. The treatment is prevention of injury to themselves or others, quiet and peaceful retirement, music, and occupation of mind. The paragraph itself is worth while having near one, in order to show clearly the medieval attitude toward the insane of even ordinarily well-informed folk, for Bartholomew was the most read book of popular information during the Middle Ages.

Bartholomew himself was only a compiler of information—a very learned man, it is true, but a clergyman-teacher, not a physician. Translations of his book were probably more widely read in England, in proportion to the number of the reading public, than any modern encyclopædia has ever been. He said:

"Madness cometh sometime of passions of the soul, as of business and of great thoughts, of sorrow and of too great study, and of dread: sometime of the biting of a wood-hound [mad dog], or some other venomous beast; sometime of melancholy meats, and sometime of drink of strong wine. And as the causes be diverse, the tokens and signs be diverse. For some cry and leap and hurt and wound themselves and other men, and darken and hide themselves in privy and secret places. *The medicine of them is, that they be bound, that they hurt not themselves and other men. And namely such shall be refreshed, and comforted, and withdrawn from cause and matter of dread and busy thoughts. And they must be gladded with instruments of music and some deal be occupied."* (Italics ours.)

Bartholomew recognizes the two classes of causes of mental disturbance, the mental and the physical, and, it will be noted, has nothing to say about the spiritual—that is, diabolic possession. Writing in the thirteenth century, diabolism was not a favourite thought of the men of his time, and Bartholomew omits reference to it as a cause of madness entirely. Food and drink, and especially strong spirituous liquor, are set down as prominent causes. It may seem curious in our time that the bite of a mad dog, or a "wood hound," as Bartholomew put it, should be given so important a place; but in the absence of legal regulation rabies must have been rather common, and the disease was so striking from the fact that its onset was often delayed for a prolonged interval after the bite, that it is no wonder that a popular encyclopædist should make special note of it.

The effect of alcohol in producing insanity was well recognized during the Middle Ages, and many writers have alluded to it. Pagel, in the chapters on Medieval Medicine in Puschmann's "Handbook," says that Arculanus, of whom there is mention in the chapter on Oral Surgery and the Minor Surgical Specialities, has an excellent description of alcoholic insanity. The ordinary assumption that medieval physicians did not recognize the physical factors which lead up to insanity, and practically always attributed mental derangement to spiritual conditions, especially to diabolic possession, is quite unfounded so far as authoritative physicians were concerned. Their suggestions as to treatment, above all in their care for the general health of the patient and the supplying of diversion of mind, was in principle quite as good as anything that we have been able to accomplish in mental diseases down to the present time. Their insanity rate, and above all their suicide rate, was much lower than ours, for life was less strenuous and conscious, and though men and women often had to suffer from severe physical strains and stresses, their free outdoor life made them more capable of standing them.

The history of human care for the insane, it is often said by those who are reviewing the whole subject briefly, may be represented by the steps in progress from the presumption of diabolical possession, and exorcism for its relief, to intelligent understanding, sympathetic treatment, and gentle surveillance, with the implication that this has all been a gradual evolution. There is no doubt that during the Middle Ages even physicians often thought of possession by the devil as the cause of irrational states of mind. Not only some of the genuinely insane—

though not all, be it noted—but also sufferers from dreads and inhibitions of various kinds, the victims of tics and uncontrollable habits, especially the childish repetition of blasphemous words, and sufferers from other psychoses and neuroses, were considered to be the victims of diabolic action. Exorcism then became a favourite form of treatment of all these conditions, but its general acceptance came about because it was so often successful. The mental influence of the ceremonies of exorcism was often quite as efficient in the cure of these mental states as mesmerism, hypnotism, psycho-analysis, and other mental influences in the modern time.

It may particularly be compared in this regard to psycho-analysis in our own day, for this cures patients by making them feel that they have been the victims of some very early evil impression, usually sexual in character, which has continued unconsciously to them to colour all their subsequent mental life. Some of the curious theories of secondary personality, the subliminal self and what has recently been called "our hidden guest," represent in other terms what the medieval observers and thinkers expressed in their way by an appeal to diabolic influence. They felt that there was a spirit influencing these patients quite independent of themselves in some way, and their thoroughgoing belief in a personal devil led them to think that there must be some such explanation of the phenomena. Even great scientists in the modern time who have studied psychic research have not been able to get away entirely from the feeling that there is something in such possession, and have admitted that there may be even alien influence by an evil spirit. The more one studies the question from all sides, and not merely from a narrow materialistic standpoint, the less one is ready to condemn the medievalists for their various theories of diabolic possession. The Christian Church still teaches not only its possibility but its actual occurrence.

Such conservative thinkers as Sir Thomas More, one of England's greatest Lord Chancellors, the only one who ever cleared the docket of the Court of Chancery, continued to believe in it nearly a century after the Middle Ages had closed, but above all is quite frank in the expression of his opinion that some of the mutism, the tics, and bad habits, and repeated blasphemies, attributed to it, may be cured by soundly thrashing the young folks who are subject to them. Neurological experts will recall similar experiences in the modern time. Charcot's well-known story of the little boy whose *tic* was the use of the word uttered by the corporal at Waterloo, and was cured by being soundly licked by some playmates at the Salpêtrière gate, is a classic. Some of the medieval cruelty represented unfortunate developments from the observations that had been made that a number of the impulsive neuroses and psychoneuroses could be favourably modified, or even entirely corrected, by attaching to the continuance of the habit a frequently repeated memory of distinctly unpleasant consequences that had come upon the patient because of it. Our experience in the recent war called to attention a great many cases of mutism, functional blindness, tremors, and incapacities of all kinds, some of which were cured by painful applications of electricity. The medieval use of the lash for such cases can be better understood now as the result of this very modern set of clinical observations.

In the meantime it must not be forgotten that the people of the Middle Ages, even when they thought of insane and psychoneurotic persons as the subjects of diabolic possession, felt themselves under the necessity of providing proper physical care for these victims of disease or evil spirits, and as we know actually made excellent provision for them. Not only were the insane given shelter and kept from injuring themselves and others, but in many ways much better care was provided for them than has been the custom down almost to our own time. They had many fewer insane to care for; life was not so strenuous, or rather fussy, as it is in our time; large city life had not developed, and simple existence in the country was the best possible prophylactic against many of the mental afflictions that develop so frequently in the storm and stress of competitive industrial city existence. This prophylaxis was accidental, but it was part of the life of the time that needs to be appreciated, since it represents one of the helpful hints that the Middle Ages can give us for the reduction of our own alarmingly increasing insanity rate.

They had no large asylums such as we have now, but neither did they have any poor-houses; yet we have come to recognize how readily they solved the social evils of poverty. The almshouses at Stratford, with their accommodations for an old man and his wife living together, are a typical, still extant example of this. Each small community cared for its own sufferers. They did not solve their social problems in the mass fashion which we have learned is so liable to abuse, but each little town cared to a great extent for its own mentally ailing. They were able to do this mainly because hospitals were rather frequent; and psychic cases were, at the beginning, cared for in hospitals, and when in milder state their near relatives were willing to take more bother in caring for them than in our time. Delirious states due to fever had not yet been definitely differentiated from the acute insanities, and all these cases then were taken in by the hospitals. This was an excellent thing for patients, because they came under hospital care early; and one of the developments that must come in our modern hospitals is a psychopathic ward in every one of them, for patients will be saved the worst developments of their affection.

The better-to-do classes found refuges for their non-violent insane in certain monasteries and convents, or in parts of monastic establishments particularly set aside for this purpose. When the patient was of the higher nobility, he was often put in charge of a monk or of several religious, and confined in a portion of his own or a kinsman's castle and cared for for years. There are traditions of similar care for the peasantry who were connected with monastic establishments, and sometimes small houses were set apart for their use on the monastery grounds. As cities grew in extent, certain hospitals received mental patients as well as the physically ailing, keeping them segregated. After a time some of these hospitals were entirely set aside for this purpose. Bedlam in England, which had been the old Royal Bethlehem Hospital for the care of all forms of illness, came to be just before the end of the thirteenth century exclusively for the care of the insane. In Spain particularly the asylums for the insane were well managed, and came to be models for other countries. This development in Spain is sometimes attributed to the Moors, but there is absolutely no reason for this attribution, except the desire to minimize Christianity's influence, even though this effort should attempt the impossible feat of demonstrating Mohammedanism as an organizer of charity and social service.

Some of the developments of their care for the insane in the Middle Ages are very interesting. Before this period closed, there was a custom established at Bedlam by which those who had been insane but had become much better were allowed to leave the institution. This was true, even though apparently there might be no friends to care for them particularly, or to guarantee their conduct or their return, in case of redevelopment of their symptoms. This amounted practically to the open-door system. The authorities of the hospital, however, made one requirement. Those who had been insane and were allowed to leave Bedlam were required to wear a badge or plate on the arm, indicating that they had been for some time in this hospital for the insane. These people came to be known as Bedlamites, or Bedlams, or Bedlamers, and attracted so much sympathy from the community generally that some of the ne'er-do-wells, the tramps and sturdy vagrants who have always been with the world as a problem quite as well as the insane, obtained possession of these insignia by fraud or stealth, and imposed on the charity of the people of the time.

It is easy to understand that wherever these patients were recognized by their badges as having been for a time in an asylum for the insane, they were treated quite differently from ordinary people. Though allowed to leave the asylum, and left, as it were, without surveillance, they were really committed to the care of the community generally. No one who knows the history is likely to irritate a person who has been insane, nor are such people treated in the same spirit as those who are supposed to have been always normal, but out of pity and sympathy they are particularly cared for. They are not expected to live the same workaday existence as mentally healthy individuals, but their pathway in life is smoothed as much as possible. Many an unfortunate incident in modern times is due to the fact that a previous inmate of an asylum is irritated beyond his power to control himself in the ordinary affairs of life by those who know nothing of his previous mental weakness. It is not unlikely that our open-door system will have to be supplemented by some such arrangement as this medieval requirement of a badge, and that we can actually get suggestions from the medieval people with regard to the care of the insane that will be valuable for us.

Another very interesting development of care for the mentally afflicted was the organization of institutions like the village of Gheel in Belgium, in which particularly children who were of low-grade mentality were cared for. This was practically the origin of what has come in our time to be called the colony system of caring for defectives. We now have colonies for imbeciles of various grades, and village systems of caring for them. At Gheel the system developed, it might be said, more or less accidentally, but really quite naturally. St. Dympna was an Irish girl-martyr whose shrine, said to be on the site of her martyrdom, existed in the village of Gheel. Her intercession was said to be very valuable in helping children of low-grade mentality. These were brought to the shrine, sometimes from a long distance, and when the prayers of relatives were not answered immediately the children were often left near the shrine in the care of some of the villagers, to have the benefit of the martyr's intercession for a prolonged period. As a consequence of this custom, many of the houses of the village came to harbour one or more of these mentally defectives, who were cared for by the family as members of it.

The religious feelings, and particularly the impression that the defectives were under the special patronage of the patron saint of the village, not only kept them from being abused or taken advantage of in any way, but made them an object of special care. They were given various simple tasks to perform, and the public spirit of the community cared for them. It was only with the development of modern sophistication that the tendency to take advantage of social defectives came and special government regulations had to be made and inspectors appointed. This system of caring for these defective children, however, was eminently satisfactory. Other villages took up the work, especially in the Low Countries and in France. The village and colony system of caring for the insane, which we are now developing with so much satisfaction, was entirely anticipated under the most favourable circumstances, and with religious sanctions, during the Middle Ages. Not a few of the defectives, when they grew up, came to be attached in various humble occupations to monastic establishments. Here they were out of the current of the busy life around them, and were cared for particularly. They were not overworked but asked to do what they could, and given their board and clothes and the sympathetic attention of the religious. There are many more of such cases at the present time than are at all appreciated. They emphasize how much of this fraternal care there must have been in the Middle Ages.

Between the village system of caring for defectives, and the germ of the colony idea in their recognition of the value of the country or small town as a dwelling-place for those suffering from backwardness of mind or chronic bodily ills that disturb mentality, and the "open-door system" for the insane, as practised at Bedlam and other places, the Middle Ages anticipated some of the best features of what is most modern in our care for mental patients. Their use of severe pain as a corrective for the psychoneuroses, even when they thought of them in connection with diabolic possession, is another striking instance of their very practical way of dealing with these patients in a manner likely to do them most good. We have had to make our own developments in these matters, however, before we could appreciate the true value of what they were doing in the Middle Ages.

APPENDIX I

Law of the Emperor Frederick II. (1194-1250) regulating the practice of Medicine.[18]

"While we are bent on making regulations for the common weal of our loyal subjects we keep ever under our observation the health of the individual. In consideration of the serious damage and the irreparable suffering which may occur as a consequence of the inexperience of physicians, we decree that in future no one who claims the title of physician shall exercise the art of healing or dare to treat the ailing, except such as have beforehand in our University of Salerno passed a public examination under a regular teacher of medicine and been given a certificate, not only by the professor of medicine, but also by one of our civil officials, which declares his trustworthiness of character and sufficiency of knowledge. This document must be presented to us, or in our absence from the kingdom, to the person who remains behind in our stead in the kingdom, and must be followed by the obtaining of a licence to practise medicine either from us or from our representative aforesaid. Violation of this law is to be punished by confiscation of goods and a year in prison for all those who in future dare to practise medicine without such permission from our authority.

"Since the students cannot be expected to learn medical science unless they have previously been grounded in logic, we further decree that no one be permitted to take up the study of medical science without beforehand having devoted at least three full years to the study of logic.[19] After three years devoted to these studies he (the student) may, if he will, proceed to the study of medicine, provided always that during the prescribed time he devotes himself also to surgery, which is a part of medicine. After this, and not before, will he be given the licence to practise, provided he has passed an examination, in legal form, as well as obtained a certificate from his teacher as to his studies in the preceding time. After having spent five years in study he shall not practise medicine until he has during a full year devoted himself to medical practice with advice and under the direction of an experienced physician. In the medical schools the professors shall during these five years devote themselves to the recognized books, both those of Hippocrates as well as those of Galen, and shall teach not only theoretic but also practical medicine.

"We also decree as a measure intended for the furtherance of public health that no surgeon shall be allowed to practise, unless he has a written certificate, which he must present to the professor in the medical faculty, stating that he has spent at least a year at that part of medicine which is necessary as a guide to the practice of surgery, and that, above all, he has learned the anatomy of the human body at the medical school, and is fully equipped in this department of medicine, without which neither operations of any kind can be undertaken with success nor fractures be properly treated.

"In every province of our kingdom which is under our legal authority, we decree that two prudent and trustworthy men, whose names must be sent to our court, shall be appointed and bound by formal oath, under whose inspection electuaries and syrups and other medicines be prepared according to law and be sold only after such inspection. In Salerno in particular we decree that this inspectorship shall be limited to those who have taken their degree as masters in physic.

"We also decree by the present law that no one in the kingdom except in Salerno or in Naples [in which were the two universities of the kingdom] shall undertake to give lectures on medicine or surgery, or presume to assume the name of teacher, unless he shall have been very thoroughly examined in the presence of a government official and of a professor in the art of medicine. [No setting up of medical schools without the proper authority.]

"Every physician given a licence to practise must take an oath that he shall faithfully fulfil all the requirements of the law, and in addition that whenever it comes to his knowledge that any apothecary has for sale drugs that are of less than normal strength, he shall report him to the court, and besides that he shall give his advice to the poor without asking for any compensation. A physician shall visit his patient at least twice a day and at the wish of his patient once also at night, and shall charge him, in case the visit does not require him to go out of the village or beyond the walls of the city, not more than one-half tarrene in gold for each day's service.[20] From a patient whom he visits outside of the village or the wall of the town, he has a right to demand for a day's service not more than three tarrenes, to which may be added, however, his expenses, provided that he does not demand more than four tarrenes altogether.

"He (the regularly licensed physician) must not enter into any business relations with the apothecary nor must he take any of them under his protection nor incur any money obligations in their regard. Nor must any licensed physician keep an apothecary's shop himself. Apothecaries must conduct their business with a certificate from a physician according to the regulations and on their own credit and responsibility, and they shall not be permitted to sell their products without having taken an oath that all their drugs have been prepared in the prescribed form, without any fraud. The apothecary may derive the following profits from his sales: Such extracts and simples as he need not keep in stock for more than a year, before they may be employed, may be charged for at the rate of three tarrenes an ounce. Other medicines, however, which in consequence of the special conditions required for their preparation or for any other reason, the apothecary has to have in stock for more than a year, he may charge for at the rate of six tarrenes an ounce. Stations for the preparation of medicines may not be located anywhere but only in certain communities in the kingdom as we prescribe below.

"We decree also that the growers of plants meant for medical purpose shall be bound by a solemn oath that they shall prepare their medicines conscientiously according to the rules of their art, and so far as it is humanly possible that they shall prepare them in the presence of the inspectors. Violations of this law shall be punished by the confiscation of their movable goods. If the inspectors, however, to whose fidelity to duty the keeping of the regulations is committed, should allow any fraud in the matters that are entrusted to them, they shall be condemned to punishment by death."

APPENDIX II

Bull of Pope John XXII., issued February 18, 1321, as a charter for the Medical Department of the University of Perugia.[21]

"While with deep feelings of solicitous consideration we mentally revolve how precious the gift of science is and how desirable and glorious is its possession, since through it the darkness of ignorance is put to flight and the clouds of error completely done away with so that the trained intelligence of students disposes and orders their acts and modes of life in the light of truth, we are moved by a very great desire that the study of letters in which the priceless pearl of knowledge is found should everywhere make praiseworthy progress, and should especially flourish more abundantly in such places as are considered to be more suitable and fitting for the multiplication of the seeds and salutary germs of right teaching. Whereas some time ago, Pope Clement of pious memory, our predecessor, considering the purity of faith and the excelling devotion which the city of Perugia, belonging to our Papal states, is recognized to have maintained for a long period towards the Church, wishing that these might increase from good to better in the course of time, deemed it fitting and equitable that this same city, which had been endowed by Divine Grace with the prerogatives of many special favours, should be distinguished by the granting of university powers, in order that by the goodness of God men might be raised up in the city itself pre-eminent for their learning, decreed by the Apostolic authority that a university should be situated in the city and that it should flourish there for all future time with all those faculties that may be found more fully set forth in the letter of that same predecessor aforesaid. And, whereas, we subsequently, though unworthy, having been raised to the dignity of the Apostolic primacy, are desirous to reward with a still richer gift the same city of Perugia for the proofs of its devotion by which it has proven itself worthy of the favour of the Apostolic See, by our Apostolic authority and in accordance with the council of our brother bishops, we grant to our venerable brother, the Bishop of Perugia, and to those who may be his successors in that diocese, the right of conferring on persons who are worthy of it the licence to teach (the Doctorate) in canon and civil law, according to that fixed method which is more fully described and regulated more at length in this our letter.

"Considering, therefore, that this same city, because of its convenience and its many favouring conditions, is altogether suitable for students and wishing on that account to amplify the educational concessions hitherto made because of the public benefits which we hope will flow from them, we decree by Apostolic authority that if there are any who in the course of time shall in that same university attain the goal of knowledge in medical science and the liberal arts and should ask for licence to teach in order that they may be able to train others with more freedom, that they may be examined in that university in the aforesaid medical sciences and in the arts and be decorated with the title of Master in these same faculties. We further decree that as often as any are to receive the decree of Doctor in medicine and arts, as aforesaid, they must be presented to the Bishop of Perugia, who rules the diocese at the time, or to him whom the bishop shall have appointed for this purpose, who having selected teachers of the same faculty in which the examinations are to be made, who are at that time present in the university to the number of at least four, they shall come together without any charge to the candidate and, every difficulty being removed, should diligently endeavour that the candidate be examined in science, in eloquence, in his mode of lecturing, and anything else which is required for promotion to the degree of doctor or master. With regard to those who are found worthy, their teachers should be further consulted privately, and any revelation of information obtained at such consultations as might redound to the disadvantage or injury of the consultors is strictly forbidden. If all is satisfactory the candidates should be approved and admitted and the licence to teach granted. Those who are found unfit must not be admitted to the degree of doctor, all leniency or prejudice or favour being set aside.

"In order that the said university may in the aforesaid studies of medicine and the arts so much more fully grow in strength, according as the professors who actually begin the work and teaching there are more skilful, we have decided that until four or five years have passed some professors, two at least, who have secured their degree in the medical sciences at the University of Paris, under the auspices of the Cathedral of Paris, and who shall have taught or acted as masters in the before-mentioned University of Paris, shall be selected for the duties of the masterships and the professorial chairs in the said department in the University of Perugia, and that they shall continue their work in this last-mentioned university until noteworthy progress in the formation of good students shall have been made.

"With regard to those who are to receive the degree of doctor in medical science, it must be especially observed that all those seeking the degree shall have heard lectures in all the books of this same science which are usually required to be heard by similar students at the University of Bologna or of Paris, and that this shall continue for seven years. Those, however, who have elsewhere received sufficient instruction in logic or philosophy having applied themselves to these studies for five years in the aforesaid universities, with the provision, however, that at least three years of the aforesaid five or seven year term shall have been devoted to hearing lectures in medical science in some university and according to custom, shall have been examined under duly authorized teachers and shall have, besides, read such books outside the regular course as may be required, may, with due observation of all the regulations which are demanded for the taking of degrees in Paris or Bologna, also be allowed to take the examination at Perugia."

Footnotes:

[1] Fordham University Press, New York, 1911.

[2] *Popular Science Monthly*, May, 1911.

[3] Philadelphia: Lippincott, 1871.

[4] The Latin lines run thus:
Si vis incolumem, si vis te reddere sanum,
 Cures tolle graves, iras crede profanum.
 Parce mero—cœnato parum, non sit tibi vanum
 Surgere post epulas; somnum fuge meridianum;
 Ne mictum retine, nec comprime fortiter anum;
 Hæc bene si serves, tu longo tempore vives.

[5] English translations of the *Regimen* were made in 1575, 1607, and 1617. The two latter were printed; the former exists in manuscript in the Library of Corpus Christi College, Oxford. The opening lines of the edition of 1607 deserve to be noted because they are the origin of an expression that has been frequently quoted since.

The Salerne Schoole doth by these lines impart
 All health to England's King, and doth advise
 From care his head to keepe, from wrath his harte.
 Drink not much wine, sup light, and soone arise.
 When meat is gone long sitting breedeth smart;
 And after noone still waking keepe your eies,
 When mou'd you find your selfe to nature's need,
 Forbeare them not, for that much danger breeds,
 Use three physicians still—first Dr. Quiet,
 Next Dr. Merry-man, and third Dr. Dyet.

[6] Some of these old medical traditions come down to us from many more centuries than we have any idea of until we begin to trace them. Ordinarily it is presumed that the advice with regard to the taking of small amounts of fluid during meals comes to us from the modern physiologists. In "The Babees Book," a volume on etiquette for young folks issued in the thirteenth century, there is among other advices, as, for instance, "not to laugh or speak while the mouth is full of meat or drink," and also "not to pick the teeth with knife or straw or wand or stick at table," this warning: "While thou holdest meat in mouth beware to drink; that is an unhonest chare; and also physick forbids it quite." It was "an unhonest chare" because the drinking-cups were used in common, and drinking with meat in the mouth led to their soiling, to the disgust of succeeding drinkers.

All the generations ever since have been in slavery to the expression that "physic forbids it quite," and now we know without good reason.

[7] The book called "The Hundred Merry Jests" suggests that the wagtail is light of digestion because it is ever on the wing, and therefore had, as it were, an essential lightness.

[8] International Clinics, vol. iii., series 28.

[9] "Historical Relations of Medicine and Surgery down to the Sixteenth Century." London, 1904.

[10] The subsequent disuse of anæthesia seems an almost impossible mystery to many, but the practically total oblivion into which the practice fell is incomprehensible. This is emphasized by the fact that while it dropped out of medical tradition, the memory of it remained among the poets, and especially among the dramatists. Shakespeare used the tradition in "Romeo and Juliet." Tom Middleton, in the tragedy of "Women Beware Women" (Act IV., Scene i., 1605), says:

"I'll imitate the pities of old surgeons
To this lost limb, who, ere they show their art,
Cast one asleep, then cut the diseased part."

[11] "Physicke is so studied and practised with the Egyptians that every disease hath his several physicians, who striveth to excell in healing that one disease and not to be expert in curing many. Whereof it cometh that every corner of that country is full of physicians. Some for the eyes, others for the head, many for the teeth, not a few for the stomach and the inwards."

[12] The Ebers Papyrus shows that special attention was paid to diseases of the eyes, the nose, and throat, and we have traditions of operations upon these from very early times. Conservative surgery of the teeth, and the application of prosthetic dental apparatus, being rather cosmetic than absolutely necessary, might possibly be expected not to have developed until comparatively recent times; but apart from the traditions in Egypt with regard to this speciality, which are rather dubious, we have abundant evidence of the definite development of dentistry from the long ago. The old Etruscans evidently paid considerable attention to prosthetic dentistry, for we have specimens from the Etruscan tombs which show that they did bridge work in gold, supplied artificial teeth, and used many forms of dental apparatus. At Rome the Laws of the Twelve Tables (*circa* 450 B.C.) forbade the burying of gold with a corpse except such as was fastened to the teeth, showing that the employment of gold in the mouth for dental repair must have been rather common. We have specimens of gold caps for teeth from the early Roman period; and there is even a well-confirmed tradition of the

transplantation of teeth, a practice which seems to have been taken up again in the later Middle Ages, and then allowed to lapse once more until our own time.

[13] Dr. Petells, discussing this use of livers (*Janus*, 1898), says that there has been some tendency to revert to the idea of biliary principles as of value in external eye diseases.

[14] "Gesammelte Abhandlungen aus dem Gebiete der Oeffentliche Medizin," Hirschwald, Berlin, 1877.

[15] See Walsh, "The Thirteenth, Greatest of Centuries," New York, seventh edition, 1914.

[16] Burdett, "Hospitals and Asylums of the World."

[17] London, 1909.

[18] To be found in Huillard-Brehollis' "Diplomatic History of Frederick II. with Documents" (issued in twelve quarto volumes, Paris, 1851-1861).

[19] Under logic at this time was included the study of practically all the subjects that are now included under the term the seven liberal arts. Huxley, in his address before the University of Aberdeen, on the occasion of his inauguration as rector of that university, said: "The scholars (of the early days of the universities, first half of the thirteenth century) studied grammar, rhetoric, arithmetic and geometry, astronomy, theology and music." He added: "Thus their work, however imperfect and faulty, judged by modern lights, it may have been, brought them face to face with all the leading aspects of the many-sided mind of man. For these studies did really contain, at any rate in embryo—sometimes, it may be, in caricature—what we now call philosophy, mathematical and physical science and art. And I doubt if the curriculum of any modern university shows so clear and generous a comprehension of what is meant by culture as the old trivium and quadrivium does." Science and Education Essays, p. 197. New York, D. Appleton and Co. 1896.

[20] A tarrenus or tarrene in gold was equal to about thirty cents of our money. Money at that time had from ten to fifteen times the purchasing power that it has at the present time. An ordinary workman at this time in England received about four pence a day, which was just the price of a pair of shoes, while a fat goose could be bought for two and a half pence, a sheep for one shilling and two pence, a fat hog for three shillings, and a stall-fed ox for sixteen shillings (Act of Edward III. fixing prices).

[21] The University of Perugia had already achieved a European reputation for its Law School, and this Papal document was evidently meant to maintain standards, and keep the new Medical School up to the best criteria of the times. The original Latin of this document, as well as of the Law of Frederick II., may be found in

Walsh, "The Popes and Science," Fordham University Press, New York, 1908. They are quoted directly from the official collection of Papal Bulls.

Notes

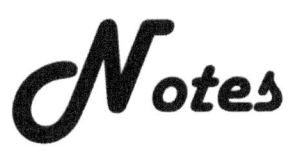

DATE: ....

Notes

DATE:

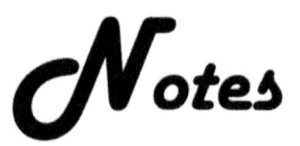

Notes

DATE:

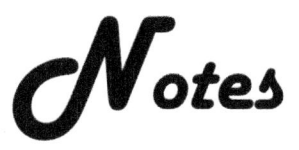

Notes

DATE: ....

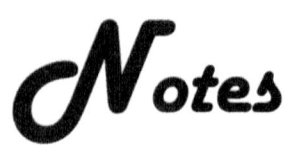

Notes

DATE:

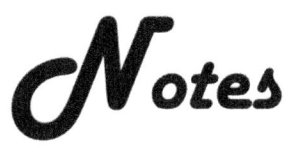

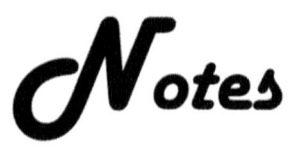

Notes

DATE:

Notes

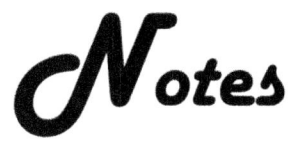

DATE:

Notes

DATE:

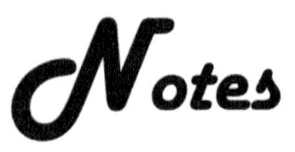

Notes

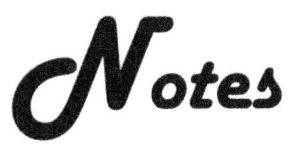

DATE:

Notes

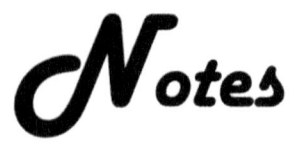

DATE:

Notes

DATE:

Notes

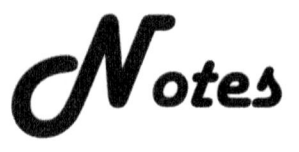

DATE: ....

Notes

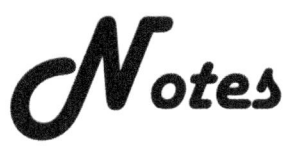

DATE: ....

Notes

DATE:

Notes

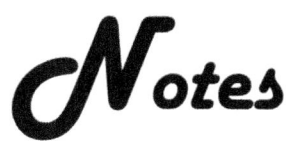

DATE:

Notes

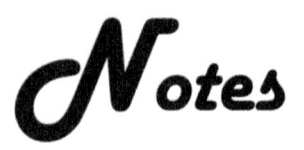

DATE:

Notes

DATE: ....

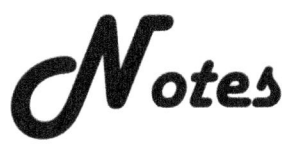

Notes

DATE:

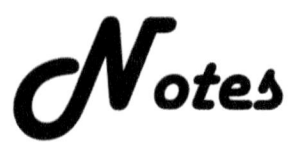

Notes

DATE:

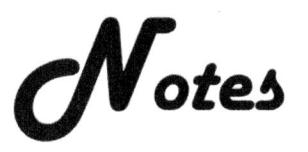

Notes

DATE: ....

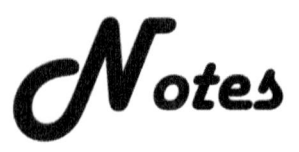

Printed in Great Britain
by Amazon